ENDORSEMENTS FOR ENERGETIC APPROACHES TO EMOTIONAL HEALING

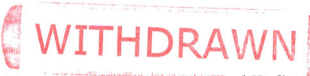

"*Energetic Approaches to Emotional Healing* offers practical and innovative methods that support and sustain health and well-being. I enjoyed it and wish you much success with this endeavor."

—Angeles Arrien, PH.D., cultural anthropologist, author of *The Four-fold Way* and *Signs of Life*

"This book effectively explores, with elegant simplicity, ways through which energy integrates spirit with mind and matter to facilitate the natural healing response."

—Leonard Laskow, M.D., author, *Healing with Love* and international lecturer

"Understanding the human being as an energy system is the new dispensation that awakens our identity to a higher level of consciousness. I honor Dorothea's work and highly recommend it to anyone interested in personal evolution."

—Jaquelyn Small, LCSW, author of *Awakening in Time, Embodying Spirit* and *Transformers*

"The book is comprehensive and practical, teaching caution and encouraging creativity." It may even convince more conservative therapists to consider alternatives when they are at an impass with traditional forms of therapy.

—Marty Wakeland, LCSW, psychotherapist in private practice

"This is the most comprehensive book on energy and psychotherapy to date–I envision it being a 'classic' primer in years to come."

—Gerry Green, MS, RN, Past President Florida Nurses' Association (FNA)

"What I love about this book is its presentation of documentation within the scientific paradigm while speaking to my heart and lifting my spirit! There is a real need for a book about healing within the context of health care. This is that book—a welcome addition to the field of energetic healing, the promotion of health, wholeness and wellness."
—Dorothy Law Nolte, Ph.D., Rolfing Instructor, author of *Children are What They Live*

"This work presents a new and innovative approach. While psychoanalysis took years, the energetic approaches presented here are effective in a few sessions."
—Phyllis Mabbett, Ph.D., RN, MFCC, Director of Behavioral Health Care Center, Scripps Hospital

"This book gives language to complex ideas and develops a meaningful ethical framework for practitioners. Thank you!"
—Gail White, Ph.D., Clinial Psychologist

"This book has been chosen to be an essential component of our new training program, Transformational Pathways, because of its comprehensive presentation of energy healing concepts and practical learning exercises. The many wonderful examples and stories bring the materials to life."
—Ruth Johnston, Ph.D., RN, Chairperson, Holistic Alliance of Professional Practitioners, Entrepreneurs, and Networkers, Inc. (HAPPEN)

Econ

Energetic
Approaches to
Emotional
Healing

DOROTHEA HOVER-KRAMER, Ed.D., R.N.
KARILEE HALO SHAMES, Ph.D., R.N.

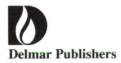

Delmar Publishers

I(T)P™ An International Thomson Publishing Company

Albany • Bonn • Boston • Cincinnati • Detroit • London •
Madrid • Melbourne • Mexico City • New York • Pacific Grove
Paris • San Francisco • Singapore • Tokyo • Toronto • Washington

NOTICE TO THE READER

Cover Design: Spiral Design
Cover Illustration: Kirsten Soderlind

Delmar Staff
Publisher: Bill Brottmiller
Production Manager: Karen Leet
Art and Design Coordinator: Carol Kechane
Editorial Assistant: Diane Biondi

Copyright© 1997
by Delmar Publishers

a division of International Thomson Publishing Inc.
The ITP logo is a trademark under license.

Printed in the United States of America

For more information, contact:

Delmar Publishers
3 Columbia Circle, Box 15015
Albany, New York 12212-5015

International Thomson Editores
Campos Eliseos 385, Piso 7
Col Polanco
11560 Mexico D F Mexico

International Thomson Publishing—Europe
Berkshire House 168-173
High Holborn
London WC1V 7AA
England

International Thomson Publishing GmbH
Königswinterer Strasse 418
53227 Bonn
Germany

Thomas Nelson—Australia
102 Dodds Street
South Melbourne, 3205
Victoria, Australia

International Thomson Publishing—Asia
221 Henderson Road
#05-10 Henderson Building
Singapore 0315

Nelson Canada
1120 Birchmount Road
Scarborough, Ontario
Canada M1K 5G4

International Thomson Publishing—Japan
Hirakawacho Kyowa Building, 3F
2-2-1 Hirakawacho
Chiyoda-ku, Tokyo 102
Japan

2 3 4 5 6 7 8 9 10 XXX 01 00 99 98 97

Library of Congress Cataloging-in-Publication Data
Hover-Kramer, Dorothea.
    Energetic approaches to emotional healing / Dorothea Hover-Kramer, Karilee Haio Shames.
        p, cm.
    Includes bibliographical references and index.
    ISBN 0-8273-8417-3
    1. Mind and body therapies. 2. Vital force—Therapeutic use. 3. Mental healing.
I. Shames, Karilee Halo. II Title.
RC489.M53H68 1997
615—dc20

                                                            96-35567
                                                                 CIP

TABLE OF CONTENTS

AUTHORS' INTRODUCTION

How would you like to deeply touch the lives of clients and loved ones with your caring? To awaken their greatest wisdom without speaking? To help them to feel better, no matter what the cause of their present discomfort?

This book is about expanding our work as caregivers through the addition of energy-oriented interventions to diminish emotional distress. The ideas presented blend well with established forms of psychotherapy, enhancing the options available for both therapists and clients. In addition, the concepts show ways of approaching emotional self-care that can have a direct impact on your personal sense of well-being, whether you are a person seeking further awareness or a health care professional.

This past century has witnessed the rise of the young science of psychology, dedicated to finding ways of assisting people with emotional distress and improving their quality of life. Perhaps in no other field is there as much controversy as in the one that deals with the complex arena of human emotions and the human soul. Freudian analysis sought to provide opportunity for the troubled mind to unburden itself. The role of the helper was, for the most part, to silently witness the individual's process, in the hope that the client would eventually be able to see his or her own life patterns and make appropriate changes through insight.

In the latter half of the twentieth century, the focus shifted to an increasingly more active therapist role. Jung's extensive writing expanded Freud's ideas, bringing dreams and images into conscious awareness and allowing for a more collaborative process between client and therapist. Many newer modalities have since sprung up, honoring the depths of the clients' imagery and the creative work of their therapists. Some of these include Gestalt therapy, bioenergetics, interactive imagery, holotropic breathwork, and deep tissue body work. All of these methods facilitate emotional release and offer an increased sensitivity to the interconnection between the psyche (mind/soul) and the soma (physical body).

Approaching the twenty-first century, public awareness has moved toward an integrated understanding of healing, honoring the fact that we are multifaceted combinations of body, mind, and spirit. This concept, understood as the *holistic* framework, allows for a multidimensional view of the client in which evolving layers of consciousness interconnect with each other. Each dimension is directly affected by the client's unique combination of heredity and environment, as well as his or her developing understanding, beliefs, and attitudes.

The holistic conceptual model, coupled with the consumer's increased ability to articulate needs, allows for an expansion of self-caring practices. In addition, there is increasing recognition for a wide variety of complementary modalities, often called *alternative approaches*. All of us in the healing and/or caring arts are continually challenged to expand our view of human nature and to understand how interconnected human beings are in intrapersonal, interpersonal, and transpersonal dimensions.

The field of counseling is moving toward a more comprehensive, integrative approach in the treatment of emotional issues. Growing in the awareness that humans need to be contacted on many levels, psychotherapy is expanding beyond the edges of predominantly linear thinking to include intuitive, creative, and spiritual aspects.

Furthermore, new explorations in molecular biology, body/mind medicine, and field theory are bringing fresh ideas and new hope into the therapeutic arena. Quantum physics, especially, seems to reiterate the mystical wisdom of ancient cultures by providing explanations such as the human energy field and the ensuing interconnectedness of body, mind, and spirit. As a result, pioneering psychologists, family counselors, research scientists, somatic therapists, physicians, and nurses are envisioning new models of human nature. The human organism is seen now as consisting not of matter, but rather of particles and waves that are mediated and influenced by human consciousness. Scientific research demonstrates what the ancients knew intuitively: the human form visible to the eye is not the whole picture, just as the actual range of sound is far more expansive than can be appreciated by the human ear.

The energy surrounding the human field interacts with the physical body, continually affecting health and behaviors. The interacting particles and waves are also in constant interplay with other people and the environment. Thus, we operate as interacting fields of energy, sharing similar properties with other energy fields. We are open systems, changing constantly as a result of input, throughput, and output of energy.

Several popular books have come forth in the last decade to demonstrate our complex, energetic nature. In 1988, Richard Gerber, M.D., wrote *Vibrational Medicine*, describing how energetic principles are rapidly developing in modern medical practice as witnessed by the MRI, lithotrypsy (for dissolving kidney stones with the use of sound waves), and the PET and CAT scans, to name only a few. In 1991, Michael Talbot published *The Holographic Universe* in which he demonstrates how the web of subatomic particles that compose our physical universe resembles a huge hologram. His book further describes ways the holographic model permits us to explain archetypal experiences, encounters with the collective unconscious, and altered states of consciousness. In 1993, Larry Dossey, M.D., commented in detail about the effects of nonlocal, noncontact energetic interventions in the best-seller, *Healing Words*. These interventions include various forms of prayer, good wishes, and heart-centered projections of human caring.

Each of these important books points to the interconnectedness among human beings. An obvious next development is to utilize this emerging knowledge for emotional healing and psychotherapy. The increasing frequency of behavioral disturbance points to the need for balancing human energies. Working with the human energy field is one way of restoring balance and harmony in individuals and environments.

This book, then, is the authors' collaborative endeavor to apply a new energy-oriented model to emotional healing. It embraces the wisdom inherent in ancient cultures and combines it with the most advanced thinking of modern science. The project ultimately develops a method for working heart-to-heart with clients and loved ones by helping to balance their energy fields. Another prominent outcome of energetic repatterning is the ability to connect with forces greater than our localized selves through the transpersonal perspective, reaching beyond the personal to the spiritual dimension.

As psychotherapists, we are committed to guiding others through the rocky terrain of psychological understanding and to shed light on motivation, choices, and actions. As nurses, we are devoted to new models of human caring. As educators of health care professionals, we are learning about subtle energies by allowing human energy fields to be our teachers. As social scientists, we envision a healthier human community through the sharing of specific knowledge and skills in energy healing.

We invite you to participate in the healing of our beloved planet and all that live here through the ideas put forth in this book!

Dorothea Hover-Kramer, Ed.D., R.N.
Karilee Halo Shames, Ph.D., R.N.

A NOTE ABOUT THE LANGUAGE USED IN THIS BOOK

The authors have done their best to clarify new or unusual concepts throughout the book, and a Glossary is available as an additional resource. Some of the terms are unique because they describe subtle energies that have not been written about before, especially in the context of emotional healing.

Throughout, the metaphor of therapist and client is used to describe the interaction between the facilitator of the energetic interventions and the recipient. The applications of the work are certainly not limited to psychotherapists and their clients; they are appropriate to interactions between colleagues, friends, and family members, as well as for self-help. Since all healing is ultimately self-healing, we might also think that everyone's internal structure contains a therapist and client, or a nurturing parent and inner child. As the concert pianist who is also a student through daily practice, there is a player and a coach within each of us.

To continue with the metaphor of client and therapist, we use a number of synonyms. The "client" is also "patient," "heelee," "receiver," and "learner." The "therapist" can be a healing arts practitioner from many disciplines—nursing, medicine, psychology, social work, case management, massage therapy, family counseling, or an allied mental health field. The synonyms we use for all of these forms of therapists are "helper," "healer," "practitioner," and "facilitator."

The ever-befuddling convention of the English language to require specific gender pronouns is resolved by using both male and female pronouns interchangeably when describing clients and therapists. Thus, for clarity, therapists are identified as masculine and the clients as feminine in some chapters, whereas the reverse is true in other chapters.

In the case examples, we have disguised the names and identifiable personal characteristics of the clients to protect anonymity. However, the patterns and their energetic resolution are accurate descriptions from numerous case files in our extensive psychotherapy practices and those of our colleagues.

ACKNOWLEDGMENTS

First of all, we would like to expressly and gratefully thank all of our content reviewers who read the entire manuscript and gave us their valuable ideas and recommendations:

Gerry Green, M.S., R.N., C.N.S
Ruth Johnston, Ph.D., R.N.
Phyllis Mabbett, Ph.D, R.N., M.F.C.C.
Dorothy Nolte, Ph.D.

Martin Rossman, M.D.
Marty Wakeland, L.C.S.W.
Gail White, Ph.D., L.C.P.
Janet Ziegler, Ph.D., R.N.

In addition, each of us would like to recognize and thank the many teachers, mentors, and colleagues who have assisted us in our healing journeys including Dr. Dolores Krieger and Dora Kunz, Barbara Dossey, Dr. Lynn Keegan, Dr. Ruth Johnston, Merla Hoffman, Sue Collins, Dr. Noreen Frisch, Heather Kussman, Joan Mariah, Jacquelyn Small, Stan and Christina Grof, Jane Hollister, Barbara and Deno Kazanis, Sheryle Baker, and Dr. Elizabeth Kuebler-Ross.

We want to thank our students and clients for sharing their lives with us and for teaching us so directly about human energy.

We also recognize the support of Delmar Publishers in bringing this project to completed form, especially with the help of Lynn Keegan, William Burgower, William Brotmiller, and Karen Leet. Cher Privett from Bakersfield, California rendered the artwork with understanding and intuitive perception.

Most definitely we wish to appreciate our enduring family members for their supportive presences throughout the project. Dorothea thanks the gentle soul of her husband, Chuck Kramer, for taming computers and holding the light. To each of her children, Anne Hover, Dr. Franz Hover, and Dr. Karen Hover "and their loved ones" goes a warm, timeless, energetic hug.

Karilee gratefully acknowledges "her healing children, Shauna, Gigi, and Gabriel, as well as Rich, the master spark in my swirling world of energetic connections" along with family members Sherry Helene Deutsch, Gloria Ingraham, and I. J. Feibus.

We conclude with acknowledgement of each other for seeing the work in different ways, thus enriching each other's process.

ABOUT THE AUTHORS

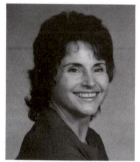

Dorothea Hover-Kramer, Ed.D., R.N., is a licensed clinical psychologist in private practice in the San Diego area. She is the author of *Healing Touch: A Resource for Healthcare Professionals* and two books of poetry. She has been active in leadership of the American Holistic Nurses' Association (AHNA) for 15 years and helped to found the Healing Touch program in 1989 as well as Transformational Pathways, a program in multidimensional healing that began in 1996.

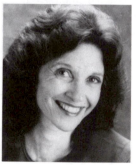

Karilee Halo Shames, Ph.D., R.N., is a clinical specialist in psychiatric nursing and a Certified Holistic Nurse practicing in the San Francisco area. She is author of *The Gift of Health, The Nightingale Conspiracy,* and *Creative Imagery in Nursing.* She is currently Director-at-Large and California Coordinator for AHNA and an instructor with the Transformational Pathways course.

Both are founding directors of the Holistic Alliance of Professional Entrepreneurs and Networkers, Inc. (HAPPEN) and are available to teach energy concepts nationwide to nurses, physicians, psychotherapists, and other health care professionals.

AN EXPANDED VIEW OF HEALING

I

*I*n our opening section, we explore the meaning of healing within the holistic context and the resulting increased interest in complementary modalities. A brief introduction to emotional healing through the human energy field follows with historical background and research findings. The next chapter gives a fascinating case example and shows ways that energy healing principles can be incorporated into a practice of psychotherapy. The third chapter continues to extend our view of healing by suggesting that rapport formation is facilitated through an interconnecting of human energy fields. The resulting synergy is enhanced through the use of intuition and intentional focusing on the part of the helping professional.

1 HEALING AS MULTIDIMENSIONAL EVOLUTION

What does it mean to be healed?
It means to become whole
To remember who we are
To reconnect with our source
To find our way home again
After a long journey.
                    —DHK

In this book we explore approaches to emotional healing that encompass energetic principles. Our working premise is that true healing is multidimensional: healing impacts all aspects of the human being to facilitate integration of the whole. If we begin with the emotional aspect, the nature of full healing will facilitate release of embedded memory or trauma, help restructure thought patterns, ease distress in the physical body, and enhance the client's sense of connection with qualities beyond localized self to the transpersonal dimension.

The word *healing* is derived from the Greek *holos* and the German *heilen*, meaning to restore to balance or wholeness. This is the root of the English words "whole," "hale," and "holistic," as well as of "healing." Specifically, the English definition of healing is "to make sound or whole," "to cause an undesirable condition to be overcome," "to restore to original purity and integrity," "to reconcile a conflict," and "to make something less grievous"(Webster, 1989).

This broad definition of healing stands in contrast to the word *cure*, which originally was listed as a synonym for healing. In current usage, however, cure means complete resolution of a physical problem by eliminating its presence with surgical excision or by chemically altering a physical imbalance. Unfortunately, few problem conditions can be resolved in such a neat and tidy fashion. The presence of chronic physical illness and enduring emotional pain, so severe that it can be a limiting factor in a client's entire life, have forced us to widen our ideas about the nature of healing.

In the vast literature of psychotherapy, the concept of healing is not yet fully accepted because it suggests something subjective, unmeasurable, and mystical. Despite the fact that the word "psychology" actually means study of the soul (the psyche), most current psychological research addresses cognitive aspects of behavior that can be measured in objective terms. Fortunately, we are living in a time of a tremendous conceptual shift toward a more holistic, integrative view. Holistic thinking allows us to define the multidimensional nature of the human being more fully and gives us a practical framework for exploring an expanded notion of healing.

THE HOLISTIC FRAMEWORK

Holistic, or integrative, approaches suggest that there are many dimensions beyond the physical for us to address in human caregiving including the emotional, the mental, and the spiritual domains. One of the major current shifts in health care is emphasized by the need for an interdisciplinary approach to client care. Clients do not come in separate, exchangeable parts like cars, despite the realities of high technology that have brought about hip replacement surgery and liver transplants. Whether there is consistent agreement or not, caregivers in hospitals must consider the physical and social environments of their patients before discharge if their interventions are to have lasting effects. Similarly, we as caregivers recognize that a client's emotions can significantly enhance or diminish the effectiveness of the most sophisticated medical interventions.

Broader concepts of psychological healing, then, must address all aspects and encompass the whole individual which is greater than the sum of separate parts. Inherent in the holistic philosophy is a wider view, one that sees healing as a process in which the individual evolves toward wholeness in as many dimensions as possible throughout his lifetime.

For instance, according to our present state of knowledge, AIDS is considered an incurable disease. However, most people with AIDS are greatly in need of healing. They may need to mend their interpersonal relationships, to resolve internal conflicts including resentments about their illness, to sense that they belong to a larger, caring universe, or to enhance their quality of life. Studies have shown that there are direct effects on the physical body's immune system with emotional counseling and resulting lifestyle changes (Hay, 1987; Jaffe, 1992). Further, an attitude of well-grounded hopefulness amplifies immune defenses and repair mechanisms.

Another aspect of healing, important in such long-term illnesses as cancer or AIDS, is the emotional support needed for the process of dying. During this time, the client needs to achieve a sense of closure in his relationships with others, to set his affairs in order, and to make peace with his higher self and his spiritual beliefs to the fullest extent possible, all in preparation for transition. Thus, we comprehend the seeming paradox, "The patient is healing while dying" when we adopt the wider, holistic definition of healing.

Holistic thinking has given us a conceptual framework for this expanded view, and with it, an understanding of the rightful place of the many alternative, complementary therapies for the care of body and mind. A large and growing literature supports application of this new paradigm in health care settings (Dossey, 1987, 1989; Weil, 1995; Keegan, 1994; Dossey et al., 1988). One example of holistic thinking and how it is permeating mainstream psychological care is evident in the rise of mind/body concepts in behavioral science, creating interdisciplinary bridges among physicians, nurses, and psychotherapists (Borysenko, 1987; Rossi, 1986). So vast is the impact of holistic thinking on all dimensions of health care in the nineties that we might correctly speak of it as a powerful and growing paradigm shift.

THE HOLISTIC PARADIGM IN PSYCHOTHERAPY

In addition to fostering changes in the practice of health care, the holistic framework has ushered in a number of emerging concepts for therapists as well. For example, the holistic approach views all symptoms, whether physical or emotional, as feedback about the nature of the whole person. This is in contrast to the concept that isolated, discrete events cause pathology, as implied in diagnostic manuals. The question is not so much *what* dysfunction the patient has, but rather *who* the client is that has the dysfunction, and *how* the symptoms are related to the client's social environment.

Further, the therapeutic alliance is no longer seen as a relationship between wise therapist and willing patient, but rather as a dynamic interaction between two human beings, one of whom has explored inner, psycho-spiritual realms and the other who is an active seeker on the path to self-discovery. Thus, the relationship is one of trust and mutual truth-telling, a partnership in which therapist and client, nurse and patient, teacher and learner, seek personal development.

Another aspect of the holistic perspective is the willingness to enlist a number of modalities for problem resolution. In therapy, this can mean considering complementary modalities rather than limiting oneself to a single approach. As most therapists are eclectic in their delivery of care, many are already making referrals for body-oriented therapies and other newly emerging modalities, including energy balancing. These various modalities are becoming an integral part of treatment planning. The effective counselor is one who can monitor all levels of the client's experience and facilitate the client's learning process.

Inherent in the holistic paradigm is a reverence for all of life, an acknowledgment of the uniqueness of each person, and an appreciation for the great diversity of the human family. Thus, a cornerstone of the holistic ethic is the building of healthy relationships with others. In the broadening, holistic context, the word "others" is not only limited to our immediate relatives and friends, but also to the global community, and beyond that to other species, animals, plants, and especially to the environment which sustains us. The well-known nursing theorist, Martha Rogers asserted, "Human beings are defined as irreducible energy fields, infinite and integral with one another and the environment. Our patterns are continually changing, innovative, and creative" (Rogers, 1987).

Such an integrated viewpoint is clearly lacking in our current health care system. For example, in a single day, a patient may seek help for arthritis from the rheumatologist; for cardiac arrhythmia from the cardiologist; for a throat infection from the internist; for education about how to take medications from the nurse or pharmacist; and for guidance about specific exercises from the physical therapist. Similarly, the counseling field offers multiple specialties for addressing diverse concerns, but the continuity needed for personal self-development may be lacking. We may, for instance, see a single client who is suffering from post-traumatic stress disorder, along with marital conflict, sexual dysfunction, difficulty with teenagers in his family, and conflict in the workplace. The best treatment approach actually may *not* be to single out one issue at a time or to refer the client to specialists. We must ask then, how could a more unified approach be accomplished? How could these various concerns be integrated to assist the distressed person to gain self-understanding?

The holistic rubric suggests looking at causative patterns, the unexpressed needs that trigger the various symptoms. Further, experience suggests that many client problems are related to embedded patterns in the individual's energy system that are repeated throughout one's lifetime until they can be brought to conscious awareness and released. The work of the energy healer is to assist clients in uncovering the underlying causes of their symptoms, as well as simultaneously inspiring their will to be well. As Betsy's story in the next chapter exemplifies, the client may have her own unique, intuitive way of moving to core issues while the therapist facilitates energetic release and allows for new synthesis.

A BRIEF HISTORY OF ENERGY APPROACHES TO HEALING

Energy can be defined simply as the vital life force that differentiates a living being from a non-living one. In the over 5,000-year-old tradition of yoga, this life force is called *prana*; in the ancient Chinese tradition it is called *ch'i*. All cultures have names for the energy or life force (Pavek, quoted in Hover-Kramer et al., 1996, p. 12) including *spiritus* in Latin, which links the idea of energy and vitality to the root of the English word "spiritual."

Healing with the concept of energy is as ancient as human history and universal cross-culturally. Shamanic approaches hold the idea that energy is brought to the suffering person through the shaman's ability to mediate between physical and spiritual realms. Throughout written history, healing knowledge has been enhanced by the helping person's unique abilities to mediate energy flow. In the past three decades, energy-oriented healing has moved forward from the metaphysical realm into mainstream health care as a viable complement, or adjunct, to other therapies.

In the early seventies, Dr. Dolores Krieger of New York University evolved a specific process for working with energy that she came to call Therapeutic Touch. The work is totally noninvasive and involves responding to cues from the client's energy field. The client is usually fully dressed while the healer uses light touch over specific body areas or in the field, depending on the needs of the healee. The words "non-contact Therapeutic Touch" have been used to describe this approach in research literature to standardize the specific maneuvers used. Over eighty colleges and universities now teach Therapeutic Touch, and it is estimated that over 30,000 healthcare professionals, predominantly nurses, have learned the concepts. Additionally, over 150 articles and academic theses have been published about this important work (Krieger, 1993).

In 1990, the American Holistic Nurses' Association developed a certificate program in energy-related healing called Healing Touch that incorporated concepts of mind/body medicine and holism. In addition, the program included ideas and techniques of other healers such as Barbara Brennan, Rosalyn Bruyere, Brugh Joy, and their many students, including Janet Mentgen, Sharon Scandrett-Hibdon, and the authors (Hover-Kramer et al., 1996, p. 27). Many other schools of energy healing are currently active, suggesting a growing interest among consumers and professionals in energy healing concepts (for a listing, see Appendix A). A comprehensive new national program of multidimensional healing, called Transformational Pathways™, has been developed by the authors and their colleagues in 1996. This program is unique in emphasizing the work of leading theorists, the principles of working with subtle energies, the transpersonal perspective, and the maturing of personal healership. The development of the healing professional is encouraged through three separate practitioner tracks: 1) nurses and other health care professionals; 2) psychotherapists and mental health specialists; and 3) somatic, or body-oriented, therapists.

While each program differs in emphasis and specific approaches, the underlying principles support the concept that healing energy moves from the fuller, focused field of the helper to the depleted, or constricted, field of the client. This flow of energy, or life force, is mediated by the healer's conscious intent to assist the client, through centering or focused alignment. Transfer or modulation of energy results in discernible changes in the client, such as deep relaxation, relief of pain sensation, lessened anxiety, and a sense of well-being. In short, work with the human energy field seems to activate energetic repatterning in the client by enhancing the inherent potential for healing in all dimensions.

RESULTS OF ENERGY-RELATED HEALING

A large and growing body of anecdotal and research accounts points to definable results from energetic interventions. Early work by Bernard Grad and associates in Toronto showed that the focused consciousness of the healer can change the molecular structure of water held in the hands (Grad, 1963). Research to measure effects of energy-oriented interventions on bacteria, enzymes, and human subjects has continued over the past three decades, and nearly 300 such projects have been listed by Daniel Benor (1990). Recently, Glen Rein conducted several experiments to establish that focused human intentionality can produce significant changes in DNA conformation (Rein, 1996). Valerie Hunt, from the University of California—Los Angeles (UCLA), showed how consciousness-mediated energy healing impacted the electromagnetic spectrum of research subjects (Hunt, 1995), and Hiroshi Motoyama and his colleagues at the California Institute of Human Sciences actually measured the human energy field, the meridians, and energy imbalance of the internal organs (Motoyama, 1993). The extensive and growing research literature from Therapeutic Touch reports significant changes in healee's anxiety states, headaches, wound healing, and sense of well-being (Quinn, 1988; Krieger, 1990). A current grant from the National Institutes of Health Office of Alternative Modalities (NIH-OAM) is providing funding to explore the effects of Therapeutic Touch on the human immune system.

As yet, very little has been written about effects of energetic approaches in the realm of psychotherapy, something we hope to remedy with the writing of this book and by citing numerous case examples. Two studies so far show the possible impact of energetic interventions in clinical settings. Gagne and Toye (1985), two Therapeutic Touch practitioners, found a reduction of anxiety in hospitalized psychiatric patients. More recently, Pamela Potter Hughes, a Therapeutic Touch practitioner and certified Healing Touch instructor, reported significant effects with a population of seven adolescent psychiatric patients. The results with these difficult, acting-out teens showed a more positive attitude, increased ability to be quiet, improved thinking patterns, and enhanced affective expressiveness. She concludes,

> When asked what they noticed about their feelings from receiving Therapeutic Touch, the adolescents reported being more calm, less hyper, happier, less agitated, relieved from tension, having more energy, a positive attitude, more courage, more control of feelings, and more ability to express feelings appropriately. [S.] noted, 'I learned about my feelings, that they can be controlled.' (Hughes et al., 1996, p. 16).

Our own experiences in working with psychotherapy clients on an outpatient basis confirm many of the results reported and go beyond the currently available research literature to show applications for a wide range of emotional distresses. We have worked with many anxious clients, including Post-Traumatic Stress Disorder (PTSD) and trauma victims, and found that they were able to achieve a deep sense of relaxation. More important, they were able to use some of the concepts later to help themselves whenever they became agitated. We have also worked with persons who were deeply depressed because of grief and chronic pain, and found that they became more responsive to their environments, more alert, and more focused after receiving energetic interventions. Similarly, we addressed energetic imbalance caused by extreme anger states, repressed emotional material, and obsessive thinking patterns, and found positive shifts to increased inner harmony and sense of equilibrium.

San Diego psychologists Gail White and Ann Carson report, "Energy work provides a powerful tool for facilitating relaxation, self-awareness, and healing from emotional wounds.

The work is complementary to other treatment modalities . . . The mind-body connection is truly evident in this work" (White and Carson, 1996, p. 9). They also describe the effects of their working energetically with anxiety disorders, panic, and post-traumatic stress. Furthermore, they have taught basic principles of energy balancing to selected patients ". . . resulting in empowerment of the patient and increased partnership in the therapy" (p.9).

We will consider psychoenergetic approaches to numerous emotional issues through various case examples in succeeding chapters.

ENERGY HEALING RELATED TO HUMAN CONSCIOUSNESS

Describing our work as *energy healing* gives the best currently available metaphor for therapeutic approaches that utilize non-contact interventions in the client's energy field. The most important factor, within our current level of understanding, is the focused consciousness of the facilitator, thus the words "consciousness-mediated energy healing" (CMEH) are relevant. Victoria Slater, an advanced student of healing theories, writes about CMEH and defines consciousness as ". . . one's multidimensional primary essence that precedes, and continues through, and [extends] beyond physical life. Its less observable dimensions can be reached through an altered state of consciousness such as in meditation, hypnosis, or centering" (Slater, 1996, p. 234).

There are obviously many theories of healing, enough to fill many volumes. For our discussion here, we will follow the concept of the transformative quality of the healer's focused awareness. The therapist's consciousness, through his intentionality, seems to assist the client by allowing new probabilities to emerge. As we consider current theories of quantum physics, we note that information is stored as an electromagnetic frequency pattern. This frequency, which contains all of the client's possible choices, can move from implicate potential, as exemplified by wave patterns, to explicate actuality, the particle form of matter, through the mediation of focused consciousness (Herbert, 1985). The healer's centering and focused intent facilitates the client's selection of more harmonious patterns from a wide sea of possibilities. It is as if the therapist's focused consciousness creates a vibrational resonance that assists the client to move toward new patterns, or higher frequencies, aligned with her unique situation.

As new patterns emerge, there may be resulting changes in the various dimensions of the human energy system. Thus, researchers are reporting changes in DNA structure (Rein, 1996) when a focused, external consciousness, such as the therapist's, is present with the distorted or impaired field of the client. Other physiological changes, such as cellular chemistry, ion exchanges, and action potentials, are also being studied (Rein, quoted in Laskow, 1992, p. 279–319). Psychotherapists report changes in emotional expressiveness, self-confidence, and thinking patterns. The client may begin to see himself and his problems from an entirely different viewpoint. For example, old limiting belief patterns such as "I am a victim of abuse" can evolve to a new perception: "I have choices; I am lovable and capable." The past experience, however painful, is no longer the only compelling force in the client's life; it may even become an opportunity for deeper compassion and understanding of others. And, as we shall explore later, many clients report a renewed interest in nurturing their souls and the spiritual dimension.

HEALING AS HEART-CENTERED CONSCIOUSNESS

Healing, then, involves a specific form of caring consciousness on the part of the therapist to achieve change toward enhanced well-being. We might recall, from a psychodynamic point of view, that all separation, whether within parts of ourselves or in relation to others, takes a tremendous amount of emotional energy to maintain. Protecting our emotional turf, old belief patterns, resentments, and things that no longer fit, is exceedingly costly from an emotional standpoint. The dissonance literally drains us. Opening to the universal vibration of forgiveness and love allows more harmony, a sense of inner balance, and attunement to inherent creativity.

Several authors of works about healing attest to the power of the universal harmonic of caring. Working with the heart center allows us, as therapists, to create an environment in which transformation of the individual can occur.

Psychiatrist Gerald Jampolsky, author of *Love is Letting Go of Fear*, states in a recent attitudinal healing brochure, "Perhaps true healing has more to do with listening and unconditional love than with trying to fix people." Nurse and leading Therapeutic Touch researcher Janet Quinn (1984) sees healing as moving into right relationship with self and others. Further, physician Leonard Laskow sees love as the powerful protective and transformational force in his work with energy-oriented healing, described in *Healing With Love* (1992). To round out our understanding, leading transpersonal philosopher Frances Vaughan writes (1995, p. 183), "The healer includes and harmonizes the opposites and brings them into balance. This archetype is associated with the fourth chakra in yoga psychology, the heart center, where the opposites intersect. A healer embodies the quality of compassion."

A majority of professionals working to help others would agree that their caring heart opens doors to understanding and empowering their clients. In this volume, we explore the intriguing ways in which the energetic heart center and the caring quality of the therapist's energy field can become the catalyst for multidimensional transformation of the client. In facilitating the balancing of the client's energy field, we embody the art of compassionate spirit.

SUMMARY

To summarize, we have begun to explore a model of healing within the context of holistic practice. Further, we have discussed the impact of the holistic paradigm and complementary modalities on the field of psychological care. This led us to consider the work of energy-oriented healing practices that have been popularized in mainstream health care for the last twenty years through the conceptual model of Therapeutic Touch and other energy-related programs.

From this, we have suggested that interventions within the human energy field are relevant to the practice of psychotherapy as well. We view emotional health as a multilevel, dynamic, and multidimensional balance within the individual. Building on the foundation of holistic thinking and the broadening definition of what it means to be healed, we now have a framework for a deeper look at increasing emotional well-being by means of energetic approaches.

In the next chapter, we explore the direct experience of this work through the eyes of our first client, whose inner adventure brought about a remarkable shift in her being.

REFERENCES

Benor, D. J. "Survey of spiritual healing research." *Complementary Medicine Research*, Vol. 4: 9, 1990.

Borysenko, J. *Minding the Body, Mending the Mind.* New York: J.P. Tarcher, 1987.

Dossey, L. *Recovering the Soul.* New York: Bantam Books, 1989.

Dossey, L. *Space, Time and Medicine.* Boulder, CO: Shambala, Press, 1987.

Dossey, B., Keegan, L., Guzzetta, C. and Kolkmeier, L.G. *Holistic Nursing: A Handbook for Practice.* Rockville, MD: Aspen Publications, 1988.; second ed. 1995.

Gagne, D., and Toye, R. "The effects of Therapeutic Touch and relaxation techniques in reducing chronic anxiety." Unpublished manuscript. Veteran's Administration, Togus, ME, 1985.

Grad, B. "A telekinetic effect on plant growth." *International Journal of Parapsychology*, Vol. 5, 1963, p. 117–134.

Hay, L. *You Can Heal Your Life.* Carlsbad, CA: Hay House, 1987.

Hover-Kramer, D., Mentgen, J., & Scandrett-Hibdon, S. *Healing Touch: A Resource for Health Care Professionals.* Albany, NY: Delmar Publishing, 1996.

Herbert, N. *Quantum Reality: Beyond the New Physics.* New York: Anchor Books, 1985.

Hughes, P.P. et al. "Therapeutic Touch with adolescent psychiatric patients" *Journal of Holistic Nursing*, Vol. 14:1, March 1996, p. 6–23.

Hunt, V. *Infinite Mind: the Science of Human Vibrations.* Malibu, CA: Malibu Publishing Co., 1995.

Jaffe, R. "Immune defense and repair systems: Clinical approaches to immune function testing and enhancement." Reston, VA: Serammune Physician's Laboratory, 1992.

Keegan, L. *The Nurse as Healer.* Albany, NY: Delmar Publishing, 1994.

Krieger, D. *Accepting Your Power to Heal.* Santa Fe, NM: Bear and Co., 1993.

Krieger, D. "Therapeutic Touch: Two decades of research, teaching and clinical practice." *Imprint*, p. 83–88.

Laskow, L. *Healing With Love.* San Francisco, CA: HarperCollins, 1992.

Motoyama, H. "Energy fields of the organism." *Life Physics.* Vol. 2:1, 1993.

Quinn, J. F. "Building a body of knowledge: Research on Therapeutic Touch 1974–1986." *Journal of Holistic Nursing*, Vol. 6, p. 37–45.

Quinn, J. "Therapeutic Touch as an energy exchange." *Advances in Nursing Science*, 6:2, 1984, p. 42–49.

Rein, G. "The in vitro effect of bioenergy on the conformational states of human DNA in aqueous solutions." *Journal of Acupuncture & Electrotherapeutics*, March, 1996.

Rogers, M. Video in *Portraits of Excellence.* Oakland, CA: Studio 3, Helene Fuld Trust Fund, 1987.

Rossi, E. L. *The Psychobiology of Mind-Body Healing*. New York: W. W. Norton & Co., 1986.

Slater, V. "Toward an understanding of energetic healing, Part I & II." *Journal of Holistic Nursing*, Vol. 13:3, Sept. 1995, p. 209–224.

Vaughan, F. *Shadows of the Sacred*. Wheaton, Il: Quest Books, 1995.

Weil, A. *Spontaneous Healing*. New York: Alfred Knopf Co., 1995.

White, G., and Carson, A. "Energy work and the mind-body connection: A path for psychologists." *San Diego Psychologist*, 5: 5, May, 1996, p. 3 & 9.

2 | BETSY'S STORY— FROM PROBLEMS TO CORE ISSUES

Two months before Christmas, a woman we named Betsy attended one of our classes on utilizing energetic approaches for emotional healing. Tears came to her eyes several times during the workshop and she asked for private counseling time. Six weeks later, Betsy and a therapist were finally able to get together one day before Christmas.

It took over two hours of travel time for Betsy to reach the office. Tears welled up before the therapist finished her usual first questions and Betsy said, "I feel like I'm on the verge of tears all the time." That's an understatement, the therapist mused.

"What makes you so sad?" she asked softly after the first flood of tears subsided.

"Lots of things," Betsy said as she described her three challenging stepchildren, aged 12, 14, and 15, whom she inherited with her second marriage three years ago. It appeared to her that the stepchildren were constantly angry about something—perhaps the divorce, perhaps their mother's hostility toward the father, perhaps the remarriage, perhaps because they were complex teenagers. The therapist made a note—*communicate with stepchildren.*

Then, Betsy described her marriage to Tom. Apparently a friendly man, he seldom set limits with the children and offered little help while Betsy floundered trying to find a way to reach them. He had never discussed feelings openly with her, but since his brother's traumatic death six months ago, he seemed totally withdrawn from his wife. Another note—*communicate with husband about traumatic death of brother-in-law.*

Next, Betsy described her job at a counseling center. Since the advent of managed care, she was only seeing half as many clients as before and instead was required to market and advertise for the organization. Her work situation was no longer satisfying in any way; in fact, she dreaded going to work. New career options were not forthcoming either; basically, she enjoyed doing individual counseling in an urban area that had an overabundance of counselors. The therapist wrote down *job dissatisfaction and career issues.*

Betsy mentioned that her only son was going to college in January. This seemed a tremendous loss to her, and she expressed more sadness. She felt that she would no longer be able to help him. Further questioning brought out that, most important, he was her major source of emotional support. Another note—*changing relationship with son.*

Now Betsy discussed her mother, a rather domineering woman who still made demands on Betsy's time and energy. "She doesn't help me much, but I can't seem to disconnect from her. She demands I call her every day. I'm overinvolved with her, and maybe with everyone else as well." The relationship with Betsy's mother was another issue for the notes.

When asked what her central issue seemed to be, Betsy declared, "I feel pressed, in the middle; I can't seem to be objective and I certainly don't have any time for myself."

No wonder, the therapist thought, looking at all of the issues that were on the list. She made a quick diagram, with Betsy in the middle, and each relationship as a pull in a different direction away from the center (see Figure 2.1).

Where does one begin with such a case? Quickly the therapist reviewed her years of training in psychological modalities that might have addressed a different aspect of the complex of issues that Betsy presented. Training in family therapy might emphasize the marital relationship and address the missing emotional communication with the husband. Experience with cognitive therapies, like transactional analysis, would lead one to look at the troublesome communication patterns with the stepchildren and explore more effective ways of interacting. Work in gestalt therapy would direct the

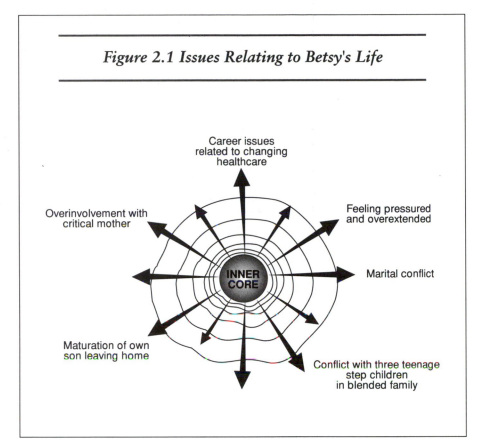

Figure 2.1 Issues Relating to Betsy's Life

therapist to look at the implied ego split that Betsy expressed: overinvolvement in the lives of others, relating to mother, son, and work issues. Intuition drew the therapist to the relationship with the son, since Betsy's emotions were most intense concerning his impending departure. Clearly, any of these paths would have led to some possible solutions and pointed at more central, core dynamics.

Since Betsy was a student of Transformational Pathways, an energy-based program, it made the most sense to begin with relaxation to assist her in finding her own starting place. The energy-oriented approach acknowledges the client's potential for self-healing, provided there is sufficient emotional support through the presence of a caring facilitator. In addition, the client's relaxed state of consciousness allows access to deeper levels of the psyche.

The therapist asked Betsy to rest comfortably in the office recliner and to release the tension and stress of her trip through relaxation breathing. She encouraged Betsy to let go of the many pressing issues for the moment, including the added pressure of Christmas time. In a few minutes Betsy's relaxation was profound, and fibrillating eye movements signified the possibility of internal imagery.

Following is a verbatim description of the therapeutic interchange as recorded by the therapist after the session.

Betsy's Story

When Betsy had relaxed, I (the therapist) asked her, "What image or memory is coming to you?"

Betsy replied, "I see my son . . . I have not done enough for him, and now it's too late to give him what I wanted to give him." She sobbed audibly as the words came out haltingly.

My rational mind was tempted to find out what she had not done for him, but I decided to stay with her image rather than to interrupt with a question. "Please see your son in front of you. And now tell me what you see," I suggested.

She looked at her son in her mind's eye and reported in a surprised tone of voice, "Well, actually he looks pretty good. He's tall and handsome, full of vim and vigor like a neat seventeen year old." There was some pride in her voice as well.

I continued, "Please look at him and notice if there is anything missing in his life right now."

"He's happy; his life is expanding and he has a great future."

"Please ask him if there's anything he needs from you right now," I suggested, wanting to make sure we had not missed anything.

"He says he's okay; I've been a good mom to him." Then her energy shifted, "But I know I haven't been a good mother." Tears started down the edge of her cheeks again.

"Well, that sounds more like an internal issue that does not seem to have much to do with your son," I responded. I wanted to help clarify the difference between the concerns Betsy might have projected onto the son and her internal, self-depreciating thought patterns. So, to complete the work in relation to the son, I suggested that she surround him with her love and, when she was ready, to release him from her awareness for the time being. One option was to see him surrounded with light, continuing to receive needed learning and resources.

While Betsy imaged this change internally, I gently helped to clear out concerns about the son by moving my hands repeatedly away from her energy field. The heaviness of her undue concern released with a seeming "pop" and Betsy felt a surge of renewed energy. The area of Betsy's energy field in which I had moved my hands now felt light and smooth.

"I feel lighter" Betsy said, as she wiggled into a more comfortable posture in the recliner. "Good," I thought. There did not appear to be any continuing attachment, which would have felt heavier and uneven to my hands. Instead, there was a clear letting go to allow the son movement toward his future. This shift was confirmed by Betsy's verbal feedback as well as by the brightening of her affect.

Now the real work at a deeper level of understanding could begin. I went on, "Feel your the energy in your body with a deep breath. Allow yourself to feel connected to your resources, the Universal Energy Field and your Higher Self."

Betsy took several deep breaths and her energy field began to feel vibrant and become fuller, except for a cool, flat area over the lower abdomen. As I felt this diminished area with my hands, I sensed we were ready to move to the subject of her feelings of inadequacy as a mother.

I continued with, "Please see yourself at an earlier time—see a younger Betsy—and go to the worst time, a time when you felt you were a terrible mother."

Betsy sorted quickly through her memory files while I moved my hands over the depleted area in her energy field above the lower abdomen.

Almost immediately Betsy had an image. It was of herself at age 21, confused, pregnant, unmarried, and trying to go to college.

"I don't like her; I don't even want to look at her. She's so disgusting," Betsy wailed.

"Please allow yourself to look at this young woman," I encouraged. "And tell me what's missing in her life. For instance, does this young woman have all the love and understanding she needs?"

Still keeping her distance, Betsy began to describe the young woman's life to me. "Well, she doesn't have any friends and her parents are alcoholics who hate each other. She does not know how to make friends so she is quick to figure out that there is some comfort in sex. She's pretty promiscuous."

As Betsy recounted the history, with obvious disdain in her voice, I mentioned in objective data "It sure makes sense that a lonely young person from a dysfunctional family would not know much about relationships."

"Yeah, but she should have known better," was Betsy's retort.

"How could she have known better? She was lonely and afraid," I offered. As Betsy persisted with her judgment of the young woman, I thought of another avenue. "Would you speak so harshly to one of your clients at the counseling center?"

"No," she admitted. "I would try to help her figure things out and make the best of the situation."

"Then do so, please," I said, while I helped to clear the congested energy over the depleted abdominal area. Betsy responded by talking to her "client," her younger self. She then explained the situation to young Betsy, helping her to see ways of dealing with her dilemma. Whenever Betsy drifted into criticism, I would stop and redirect the proceedings. Otherwise, Betsy's explanations were clear, to the point, and, most important, kind.

I then encouraged Betsy to be more specific about the future. "Please tell the young woman that she is going to do well, her son is going to become a responsible young adult, and she will become a compassionate counselor because of her experience."

When Betsy started to tell the young woman about these things, she wept and remarked, "Actually she didn't do too badly. Her life turned out rather well. Maybe she's not so disgusting after all."

"I would say rather gutsy." I suggested, "Going to college while raising a child as a single parent, learning how to build relationships, and finding a satisfying career—those sound like pretty courageous things for a young person to do."

The next step, increasing the bonding with the dissociated part of herself, required further work. When I proposed that she might want to hug the young woman, Betsy recoiled, "I would have to admit I was wrong and that there was something wrong with the family of origin."

"Yes, your family was very troubled," I agreed. "But the price you pay for being so hard on yourself is high as well. Think about how you've been feeling and how you see the issues around you. Overinvolvement may be a way of distracting yourself from the real inner pain you feel."

While she thought about this, I helped to release more of the pain, which felt like a constriction, by brushing my hands away from Betsy's energy field.

"I guess I could learn to like her," Betsy started. "She isn't perfect, but then neither were her parents. I don't have to maintain that lie to please them anymore."

I encouraged Betsy to surround the young woman with light, caring, and understanding, and to begin to feel herself embracing her dissociated younger self. As she did so, tears rolled down the sides of her face and her energy field under my hands became very warm. The flush of her face let me know that there was a deep subconscious response with activation of the autonomic nervous system.

The energy field now felt full and smooth over the entire abdominal area. I continued to hold my hands in the area to allow the final integration and reconnecting to occur.

After a few minutes Betsy opened her eyes. "I had no idea that all that was in there," she commented. "I feel like I'm more together now."

I encouraged Betsy to walk around and feel the flow of energy in her body. She sensed a renewed vitality in all parts of her being. She began to dance and sing, celebrating the joyous reconnection as if it were with a lost friend. Most important, there was a deepening respect for herself, gained through the willingness to re-experience her difficult past. Clearly, this was a dramatically different Betsy from the person that had arrived just an hour before.

When she departed, Betsy scheduled a follow-up appointment and paid me. She expressed her appreciation for the many insights. We had covered vast inner territory, something that might have taken months with more traditional therapeutic approaches. "I feel whole, healed, like I have never felt in my entire life." She smiled as she walked to her car in the sunshine.

As we reflect on this session, and many other similar hours, it is clear that this kind of integrative work is more of an art than a science. Somehow, all of the therapist's varied training courses and counseling experience came together in being fully present with Betsy. In addition, knowledge of the human energy field gave her an immediate awareness of sensing Betsy's energy flow and the areas of the field where the energy was depleted or constricted. With this added resource, Betsy was able to access an unresolved but basic and central issue—the dissociated, conflicted part of herself—very rapidly. Sensing the energy in the depleted area over the abdomen, the therapist was able to work with Betsy and guide her internal process in an unobtrusive and supportive way.

The outcome was surprising and rewarding for both of them, a tribute to the great flexibility of the psyche in finding its own solutions. Understandably, there was more work to be done, and several sessions followed this initial one with Betsy. The basic work, of getting to a core issue from a confusing array of identified problems, however, was opened in the very first hour of therapy.

SUMMARY

It is our purpose in this book to explore our understanding of the human energy system and ways of utilizing this information to assist with the therapy process. In the chapters that follow, we further describe the interventions used with Betsy and other clients from an energetic perspective and explore the underlying conceptual model. Subtle energies and their implications for supporting healthy and productive life changes offer new perspectives for multidimensional healing in the counseling world.

3

RAPPORT AND INTUITION: FOUNDATIONS OF HEALING INTERACTIONS

RAPPORT AS SYNERGY

As we look at the interactions described in the previous chapter, we note that there is a helpful interconnection between the client and the therapist. In traditional psychotherapeutic language, we call this *rapport*, the kind of bonding and trust that allows an exchange of information on a deeper than social level.

Rapport is confirmed when a client opens with a strong expression of feeling, as Betsy did. It is skillfully maintained by the therapist through constant awareness of nuance, the slightest pause or hesitation, and the unspoken elements of a conversation. If rapport or a sense of trust is missing, the finest interventions will go flat, or worse, may offend the client and impair the acceptance of further help. Such fruitless encounters may last only for one session in these days of "therapy-wise" clients, or perhaps proceed for years with mumbled references to "making progress." No matter how hard both parties try, no new ideas or proposed solutions can be fruitful if rapport is missing.

When we look at rapport as an energy exchange, we enhance our understanding of this essential foundation for all helping endeavors. If we assume for a moment that each individual is an energy field extending beyond the physical body, we might say that there is an attunement of the two energy fields. If the blending is favorable, we consider it to be harmonious and positive—a synergy. If the connection is aversive, we commonly use words such as "lack of rapport," "disharmony," or "bad vibrations" to describe the relationship.

While we have used the idea of rapport in counseling settings for decades, the idea of understanding synergy from an energy field perspective is quite new. It often appears that what is really communicated in a therapy session extends far beyond the spoken word and includes the caring presence of the helper. Some quality, the relative health and integrity of the healer's energy, seems to "rub off" and assist the client in feeling supported, encouraged, and, therefore, to look at new solutions.

Conversely, it is also apparent that helping professionals are significantly impacted by their clients' energies. For example, working with predominantly depressed patients can result in increased depression in the healer. It is not so much that the client transfers a negative quality, but that the client's depressive vibrational pattern resonates with and triggers the therapist's own tendency toward depression. Since we are all human and limited in some way, it is quite likely that a client's pattern can affect the therapist, especially if the therapist has a similar issue. This taking on of the client's pattern contributes to helper "burnout," and is a major concern for all who work in the health care field.

A catch phrase learned in professional training points to the pervasiveness of the energetic exchange between client and therapist: "either the client improves or the therapist gets worse." Something of the interchange of energy between client and practitioner—the synergy—allows clients to improve by being in the presence of a more balanced person. On the other hand, if the helper is not adequately prepared, she may begin to vibrate with an energy pattern that is similar in the client.

The resonance between the client and therapist's energy fields that we call synergy, or rapport, is enhanced by conscious attunement. The therapist chooses to tune into the client's vibrational pattern without giving up her own identity or strengths. Akin to an experienced ensemble musician, she finds the notes that allow her to play in the same key as the client, thereby creating a harmony. In ancient traditions, the shaman, or community therapist joined himself intuitively with the patient to find the best means of relieving the illness; to help his tribe, he could also become one in his mind's eye with a herd of buffalo to determine the best place for hunting.

To understand such resonance more fully, let us turn to the energy-oriented therapies taught in programs such as Therapeutic Touch, Transformational Pathways, and the Barbara Brennan School of Healing Science (and others listed in Appendix A). Here we have a framework that allows us to understand attunement, energetic interchange, and transformation more fully.

THE PRESENCE OF ENERGY FIELDS

For at least a hundred and fifty years, science has presumed the presence of energy fields to explain the influence of one object or particle on another even when they are spatially separate. This has been called the *force field* of the object, a phrase coined by the English scientist, Faraday. One form of a force field becomes visible when working with magnets. As you place a bar magnet on a paper with small iron filings around it, the filings will move away from the middle of the magnet toward the two ends, especially toward the northern end of the magnet (which points toward the earth's magnetic north pole). Since the advent of space travel, the layers of the earth's atmosphere, and the vast electromagnetic field that extends beyond our planet for several hundred miles, have become detected by radio receivers and visible to our eyes through enhanced photographic processes.

Many species of animals communicate in complex ways through their electrical or magnetic fields. For example, fish have various forms of "strong" or "weak" electrical energy. "This faculty enables them to detect the rough shape, conductivity, and location of nearby objects, recognize members of their own species, call their mates, find their position in a school, and enact other behaviors critical to their survival" (Wickelgren, 1996, p. 32). Furthermore, researchers at a number of major universities are studying magnetite and other cellular substances that serve as communication tools and inner compasses for bees, microbes, and marine mammals. Human magnetite crystals, located in the brain, may also serve as communication tools and as protection from the subtle influences of the environment. Although the implications for human health have not been fully studied, "The implication is, of course, that fields from power lines, cellular telephones, magnetic resonance imagers, and other devices could indeed be affecting people" (Kirschvink, quoted in Wickelgren, 1996, p. 37).

The impact of electromagnetic fields on the human body seems to be subtle, but pervasive. For example, some studies indicate that children living near high tension wires have an increased rate of leukemia and other cancers. The possible effect of portable telephones and other extremely low frequency fields (ELF) is currently under investigation. Even our seemingly friendly electric blankets and waterbed heaters put out low levels of electromagnetic emission that may cause cellular molecules and chromosome structures to change or mutate. Though the data thus far is not conclusive, this possibility is not so far-fetched when we consider that over one third of our daily lives is spent in bed in an altered state of consciousness, leaving us more vulnerable to such effects than in our more defended waking state.

As an aside, it is interesting to note that when Therapeutic Touch was introduced into hospital settings in the seventies, many persons were highly skeptical about the idea of energy fields and other unseen phenomena. In the nineties, however, we find that professionals and lay persons alike are intrigued by the concept of energy fields and their effects because they have already heard so much about them in the popular media.

The human energy field is much more subtle than that emitted by home appliances or computers, but it also can be measured by developing technologies. Hiroshi Motoyama, a well-known Japanese researcher, has been assessing the human energy field and major energy centers since the early 1980s with his AMI device (Gerber, 1988, p. 186–187) showing that human beings are indeed much more than physical bodies. His research also bears out what many physicians have noted during diagnostic examinations: the area around the human body is full and expanded in a physically healthy and emotionally vital person, whereas it is depleted, diminished, or constricted in someone who is physically ill or emotionally depressed (Motoyama, 1984, p. 259). Currently, Dr. Motoyama is continuing his research to bring his concept of "energy medicine" into reality through the development of high technology devices that measure human energy meridians and energy vortices. This work is being explored extensively at the California Institute of Human Studies in Encinitas (personal communication, April, 1996).

For over twenty-five years, researchers, predominantly in the discipline of nursing who studied Therapeutic Touch, have documented data about the human energy field (Krieger, 1993; Quinn, 1993). While the healthy human energy field is full, vibrant, symmetrical, and smooth to the hands of the person who does an energetic assessment, the ill person's field may be bumpy, rough, diminished, asymmetrical, or irregular in shape. Practitioners of other healing modalities also notice the same effects and use a variety of specific interventions to bring the energy field to improved balance and symmetry (Hover-Kramer, 1996).

It appears more and more clear, then, that human beings are organized energetically. As we shall learn, there is a discernible biofield extending beyond the physical body. In addition, there are energy flow pathways, called meridians, and distinctive centers of consciousness. The discipline of nursing, a strong leader in exploring the holistic nature of healing, recognizes "energy field disturbance" as an identifiable nursing diagnosis. Energy field disturbance (1.8, NANDA, 1994, p. 37) is defined as "A disruption in the flow of energy surrounding a person's being which results in a disharmony of the body, mind, and/or spirit." Defining characteristics of the diagnosis include assessment of subtle temperature differences, visual and auditory cues, disruption of the field, and patterns of movement in the flow pattern of the field. The energy field diagnosis has become the basis for energy-related interventions in mainstream nursing practice. Its presence underscores the rapid evolution of energy-oriented thinking in health care.

The implications of energy dynamics in psychotherapy are just beginning to be explored. Because all therapists consider rapport to be an important mental idea, our energetic framework suggests that rapport is a noticeable interaction between the energy fields of the healer and healee. The connection with the therapist becomes the temporary human bridge for the client to access his own resources and higher power. Another way therapists work energetically is by reaching beyond the client's story, and his temporary identification with it, to address the intent behind it. The client is seen as temporarily manifesting repeated dysfunctional patterns that can be resolved and restructured.

As therapists, we often may have spoken of sensing emotional blocks in our clients, but now we come to actually understand the blinding force of criticism, fear, guilt, and shame as impediments to the client's energy flow. Emotional distress seems to be literally encoded in the physical body as a form of cellular or holographic memory. The release process that we describe in Chapter 7 includes clearing out the embedded pattern and allowing a newer, more evolved self-concept to form.

Most therapists know that there are discernible physical effects when strong emotions are expressed. We know the healing power of crying and venting long-held emotions. Physiological changes, however, such as lowered pulse, blood pressure, and breathing rate have been repeatedly measured with energetic interventions such as Therapeutic Touch (Quinn, 1993), even when the content of emotional material was outside the client's awareness. It appears that the human energy field can move to its own balance when receiving an energetic intervention, such as modulation, without full cognition. This could be exceedingly useful in working with persons who cannot recall specific trauma or who need to discharge repressed childhood events that occurred before they were able to speak.

AWAKENING INTUITION

In counseling, we have learned that intuitive sensing is as valuable as cognitive activity. Undervalued in the medical arts, intuition is nonetheless one of the greatest skills we can share with our clients. The healer can take her full self, including her inner guidance, into every therapeutic encounter. This conscious focused intent, called *centering*, allows for maximal effectiveness in the interaction.

One of the most prominent minds to value intuitive thinking was the great psychologist Carl Jung. He suggested that intuition is neither as mystical nor as undefinable as many people have believed. Throughout his life he experienced seemingly nonlinear, acausal events that he came to call "*synchronicities*"—unusual circumstances that defied logic and yet made sense later on in his life (Jung, 1963). He came to describe intuition as a highly attuned state of being that allowed for complementary interaction of all the senses. When the therapist is intuitively seeing, feeling, smelling, tasting, and hearing, he becomes attuned to more subtle levels of existence, ones that have been accessed by musicians, writers, mystics, and spiritually sensitive individuals throughout time.

Therapy is a synergistic interaction in which the healer's intuition serves as the link to the client's subconscious aspects. "Awakening intuition is not so much a matter of gaining a skill as of removing the impediments to the natural expression of an innate human ability" states the well-known medical intuitive Caroline Myss (quoted in Leviton, 1995, p. 28). Intuition, thus, can be seen not so much as an unusual talent but as a natural by-product of the therapist's mature self-esteem and wisdom.

Intuitive insights often come quickly and spontaneously providing creative ideas, images, or unusual solutions. In therapy, they can be invaluable for allowing us to connect with deeper parts of the client's experience. Finding a balance between what we can know and what must be inferred, however, is crucial. Intuitive work does not imply abandoning reason; rather, it means a willingness to stretch our vision to what we sense even when it has not yet been proven. Working between the known and the inspired can greatly enhance our perceptive skills, surpassing knowledge that is available to the intellect alone. It is reported, for example, that Einstein imaged the famous formula equating matter and energy in an intuitive flash after traveling in his mind's eye on the end of a light beam. Undaunting scientist that he was, he took ten long years to prove the formula in mathematical terms.

ADDRESSING THE INNER SKEPTIC

As we speak of energetic approaches in psychotherapy, we need to extend our awareness to what is not yet fully explained or understood but can be grasped intuitively. The personal skeptic that allows for careful discernment is a valuable ally. It can, however, limit exploration of new arenas, such as the framework we are proposing. One way to circumvent limitations of our vision is to use an "as if" frame, trying out new concepts in a provisional manner until they are confirmed and validated by personal experience.

Marty Rossman, M.D., director of the Academy for Guided Imagery, describes his way of working with inner skepticism in the following manner (personal communication, April 19, 1996):

As a physician who has been deeply involved in traditional acupuncture, the holistic paradigm, alternative medicine, energy medicine and the like for 25 years, I confess that for many years I practiced acupuncture 'as if' there was a field of energy as described by the ancient Chinese. I figured that they were onto something that worked, even if the explanation was 'wrong' or 'partial,' and until we know better, it made sense to operate as if that's the way it worked. And of course, it does tend to work that way. About 15 years into it, I started to actually believe that *Ch'i* was real, that the energy fields existed as described, and began to work more directly with the energy fields in term of imagery, hands-on healing, and acupuncture. Most of this time, I would say I believed in *Ch'i* every other day or so. Now, I would say that I believe in it most days, but am still uncomfortable talking about it as strictly 'energy flow.' I continue to wonder about energy flow in terms of neurotransmitters, nerve transmission, peptide molecules, states of muscle tension, etc., not because either one is 'the way it is,' but in an attempt to integrate what I have perceived looking at the same phenomena from different perspectives.

Perhaps each of us has different ways of learning and integrating new ideas, and these need to be respected and acknowledged. Some of us seem to learn incrementally, gathering bits of knowledge in small amounts and trying them out, whereas others seem to grab an understanding in large chunks.

The authors had many interesting discussions about bringing energy concepts into day-to-day awareness. Dorothea learned to trust the presence of a Universal Energy Field in the days of saturation bombing of Berlin, her home when she was a child. Each morning she awoke to the gift of life supported by a mysterious force while others died in great numbers around her. She then transferred her fervent wish for healing or dying, whichever was best, to homeless animals by connecting to this energy source. This seemed to bring about good results with the animals and gave her a sense of peacefulness. The work with energy-related healing as an adult flows naturally from these early experiences, and there has never been any doubt about the effectiveness of aligning with Higher Energy.

For Karilee, the process has been a lifelong journey of growth and exploration. It began very early, when she learned to build a protective barrier around herself in the midst of family chaos. Her most significant memory occurred at age fifteen, when her mother attempted to strike her during an attack of rage. There had been many such episodes, but this time, Karilee felt more inner strength and protection. The mother's arm came down on Karilee's lower arm as she lifted it to protect her head. In her mind, Karilee was fully surrounded by a light, a sense of warmth and protection. As the mother reached her, she felt nothing. The mother, on the other hand, doubled over in pain and fell writhing to the floor. The mother's arm was broken; the teenager was unharmed. At that point, Karilee felt there was a force or field around her that prevented injury. Despite many other intuitive experiences over the years, Karilee attests to the fact that her process has been one of believing, then wondering, trusting and doubting, and remembering and forgetting. She acknowledges that this process is similar to her learning style; she often gains information, then must reaffirm her knowledge through frequent validation. The energetic model has been consistently confirmed in her work with hundreds of clients, yet she is always surprised at the results.

We have discussed the questions of skepticism and belief many times in our ongoing seminars with psychotherapists. For the most part, the group agrees that initially there needs to be a leap of faith to achieve an intuitive grasp of the energetic model. Gradually, validating experiences become more convincing as the energetic model clarifies and supports direct experience with clients. We have also come to agree that the energy field model is at best a useful working construct, based on current knowledge and the emerging concepts of quantum physics. It may well be replaced by a more comprehensive way of looking at human interactions in the future.

SUMMARY

In this chapter, we have explored the underlying foundation of rapport and intuition in therapeutic interaction. If we see rapport as a synergy between two energy fields, we understand how resonance from the higher vibrational frequency of the intentional therapist can enhance well-being of the client's field. We have also considered the scientific parameters behind energy field model and the nursing diagnosis of "energy field disturbance" as a working precept. Use of our intuitive capacities allows us freedom to consider the energetic model and to notice confirming experiences while maintaining balance with healthy skepticism.

In the next section, we explore our working model more fully, considering various aspects of the human energy field, the specific energy centers, and ways of assessing them for the planning of therapeutic interventions.

REFERENCES

Gerber, R. *Vibrational Medicine*. Santa Fe, NM: Bear & Company, 1988.

Hover-Kramer, et al. *Healing Touch*. Albany, NY: Delmar, 1996.

Jung, C. G. *Memories, Dreams, Reflections*. New York: Pantheon Books, 1963.

Krieger, D. *Accepting your Power to Heal*. Santa Fe, NM: Bear & Company, 1993.

Leviton, R. "Unraveling the biography in your biology." Intuition, 1:4, 1995, p. 26–31.

Motoyama, H. *Theories of the Chakras*. Wheaton IL: The Theosophical Publishing House, 1984.

Myss, C. *Anatomy of the Spirit*. New York: A Harmony Book, 1996.

North American Nursing Diagnosis Association, *NANDA Nursing Diagnoses, Definitions and Classification 1995–6*. Philadelphia, PA.

Quinn, J., and Strelkauskas, A. "Psychoimmunologic effects of therapeutic touch on practitioners and recently bereaved recipients: A pilot study." *Advances in Nursing Science*, 15:4, 1993, p. 13–26.

Wickelgren, I. "The strange senses of other species." *IEEE Spectrum*. March, 1996, p. 32–37.

II THE NATURE OF HUMAN ENERGY

*I*n this section, we explore human energy patterns to prepare our understanding of the emotional healing work described in the next section. We explore the dimensions, or layers, of the human energy field, the specific energy centers with emphasis on their psychological significance, and the ways that we can assess the energy field and centers by using our intuitive, higher sense perceptions. Specific exercises for centering, meditating on the energy centers, and increasing higher sense perception are included.

4 | THE HUMAN ENERGY FIELD

The human energy field, as previously mentioned, is subtle. It is only recently that technology has advanced to the point of being able to measure the energy centers and the energetic flows known as meridians. Knowledge of the human force field, however, has been conceptualized for thousands of years. As far back as recorded history, sensitive individuals have reported seeing the *aura*, the name given the human energy field in ancient texts.

For example, stone relief carvings of Egyptian temples, built over five thousand years ago, depict individuals accompanied by their *ka*, or etheric double (Hover-Kramer, 1993). Beyond the *ka*, the early Egyptians distinguished at least four other layers that extended beyond the physical body, each one finer than the previous one and reflecting progressively higher levels of consciousness (Masters, 1991, p. 19-40). Each of these layers was believed to influence intuitive powers and to assist in healing during one's lifetime and in transporting one to the afterlife. The symbol for the 'breath of life," the *ankh*, was frequently depicted as allowing the transfer of energy directly from exalted deities to humans.

Religious art abounds with pictures of the human aura, especially around the head of a gifted teacher. Halos are depicted cross-culturally and throughout the ages to identify powerful persons such as healers, saints, and shamans. Could it be that artists are actually describing what they see, not just figments of their artistic imaginations? Evidence supports the universal viewpoint that intuitive persons and artists sense the energetic emanations that are prevalent around evolved, spiritual individuals.

Mother Theresa's energy field, for example, seems to envelop and change a whole community such as Calcutta. Persons who have seen and met this living saint forget her small, fragile physical presence, and sense the grandeur of her devotion to higher service. The effect of her powerful field was in evidence while she was hospitalized in San Diego in 1994. Much to their surprise, a number of physicians found themselves agreeing to staff clinics in Mexican border towns while she was in their care. It seemed as if Mother Theresa's energy field connected with a subconscious, altruistic aspect of the doctors. To use our energetic language, her field created a resonance that lifted the vibrational pattern of those around her to a higher level. As Mother Theresa embodies the healing archetype, she connects those around her with their own sense of higher purpose.

Currently, many teachers with highly developed intuitive skills have described the human energy field. Each healer seems to "see" the energy field in a distinctive way. Barbara Brennan's beautiful book, *Hands of Light*, depicts seven layers of the energy field in vivid color and detail, as she perceived them and as interpreted by her artist (Brennan, 1987). Dora Kunz, who has been a clairvoyant intuitive since birth, describes her perceptions of the energy field in *The Personal Aura* quite differently (1993). Also noteworthy is the intuitional skill of Rosalyn Bruyere who is a powerful teacher of many healers. She researched the human energy field at UCLA with Dr. Valerie Hunt. They found that the colors produced by a meditating subject could be sensed through clairvoyance. The wave frequency patterns, associated with the colors emitted by the subject, were also simultaneously registered and recorded by electronic instrumentation (Hunt, 1995; Bruyere, 1989).

LAYERS OF THE HUMAN ENERGY FIELD

We will integrate the information from many healing practitioners to highlight those most pertinent for our present discussion. As we have experienced in teaching sessions, the first four layers of the energy field are quite easy to sense with the hands after some practice. The outer layers, however, are less pronounced and ever finer in quality. Together, the layers constitute the protective field that seems palpable when we are in the presence of a vibrant, lively individual.

First is the *etheric layer*, a structured, light blue layer that extends beyond the physical body about 1–3 inches. It is the layer that affects the physical body most directly and is therefore most relevant to physical healing endeavors. The texture of this layer is smooth with fine vertical line patterns. Next is the *emotional layer* that reflects our feeling, affective energy; it is quite fluffy, diffuse in shape, and colorful. A single color, such as red or brown, may predominate in the presence of a strong emotion such as anger or fear. The *mental layer*, called the *causal* in some texts, is smooth and more structured. It appears yellow to most sensitives, has fine vertical lines, and is supported by the individual's thought patterns. Fourth is the less structured, flowing *intuitive layer* that holds our sense of connection with dimensions beyond personal identity, perceiving ourselves as part of a greater, transpersonal Universe.

The next three layers of the field are more subtle and represent physical, emotional, and mental patterns of the individual at a higher frequency of development. The fifth layer, sometimes called the *etheric template*, is the blueprint, or underlying structural pattern, for the physical body in its fullest potential of health and wholeness. The sixth layer represents the emotions in their most developed state as a pure, unconditional vibration of Love. Finally, the seventh layer constitutes the blueprint of the soul in its highest form. It is activated when we connect with our innermost sense of purpose, the sacredness of life itself, and the divinity of our being.

If we look at the multidimensional human energy field, we see a radiant being of light as represented in Figure 4.1. The field can be considered a protective envelope of electromagnetic energy. We do not so much *have* a field; more correctly, we *are* a vibrant field.

If you are a health care professional, you may be quite inspired to see your clients as multidimensional beings, complex and beautiful, with the potential for fully developed, vital energy. This offers a healthy alternative to viewing someone as a case, a diagnosis, or a condition.

Each of us can benefit by seeing ourselves, and the persons with whom we interact, as energetic beings, as multilay-

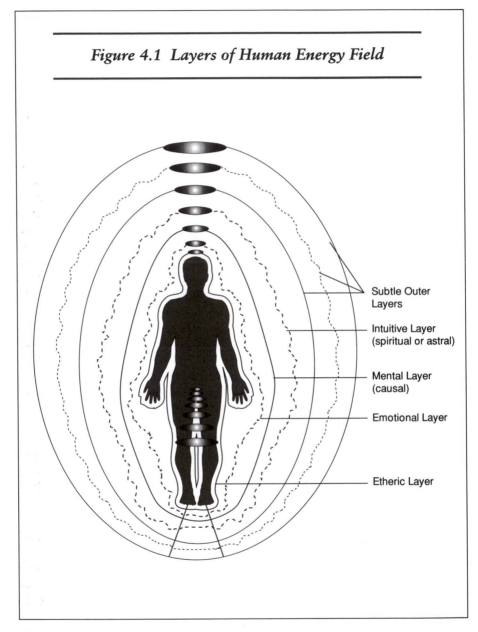

Figure 4.1 Layers of Human Energy Field

Subtle Outer
Layers

Intuitive Layer
(spiritual or astral)

Mental Layer
(causal)

Emotional Layer

Etheric Layer

ered unities. We know intuitively that we are potentially much more than our physical bodies, our emotions, or even our thoughts. We could best be considered to be finely developed spiritual beings who are having a temporary human experience. Developing scientific and intuitive knowledge of human energy fields supports this perception.

INTERACTION OF ENERGY FIELDS

Let us look at what occurs when two human energy fields begin to interact with each other. If we understand the field concept correctly, every interaction has an influence on the parties involved. Knowledge of the human energy fields makes it possible to be very conscious about our transactions rather than to be at effect, wondering what hit us on days when nothing seems to go right. For instance, if we as helping professionals walk into a family counseling setting with our centered, expanded fields, we may help to shift the energy in the room, as in the example of Mother Theresa's pervasive influence. If we face an emotionally-charged gathering without preparation, we may find ourselves feeling drained, tongue-tied, or unable to supply creative solutions.

Persons with emotional problems, such as depression, will usually have significantly depleted or constricted energy fields, as we will discuss further in succeeding chapters. To be effective, the helper must pay careful attention to her own field prior to and during a therapeutic session. The ideal quality is one of empathy, concern, and compassion, without over-involvement. This is distinguished from sympathy, where the helper may personally begin to feel the client's distress.

From an energy-oriented viewpoint, empathy and sympathy differ markedly. In empathy, the two fields are separate, with the fuller, more developed field of the helper standing firm in the face of the client's more diminished field (see Figure 4.2). There is potential here for the client's field to expand, gradually matching the therapist's, through mutual resonance. Sympathy, on the other hand, is a meshing of the two fields with energetic bands connecting the two fields. There can be no inflow of new energy in this situation. The signs of unhealthy overinvolvement are represented energetically in Figure 4.3.

There are life stages when the sympathetic energy connection occurs naturally. "Being in love" is one of the most confusing in our culture. Many poems and love songs celebrate this form of energetic enmeshing. The condition of being blindly in love, however, usually passes in a few months and

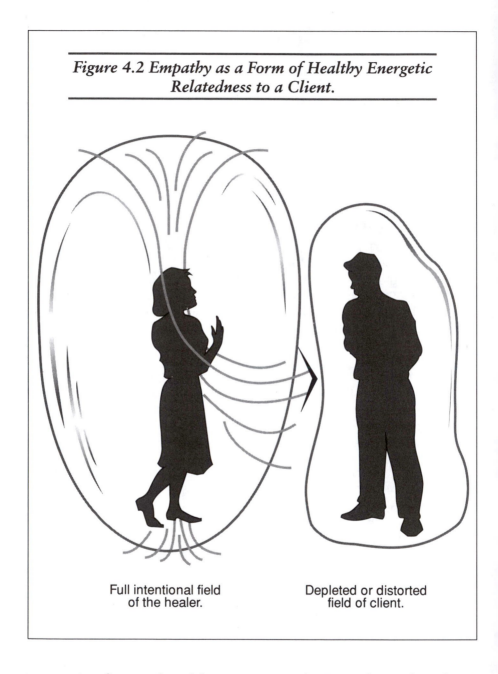

Figure 4.2 Empathy as a Form of Healthy Energetic Relatedness to a Client.

Full intentional field
of the healer.

Depleted or distorted
field of client.

is often replaced by a growing, lasting relationship that is more balanced and equal. In fact, the mark of healthy adult relationships is in the flexibility of energetic exchange. Some-

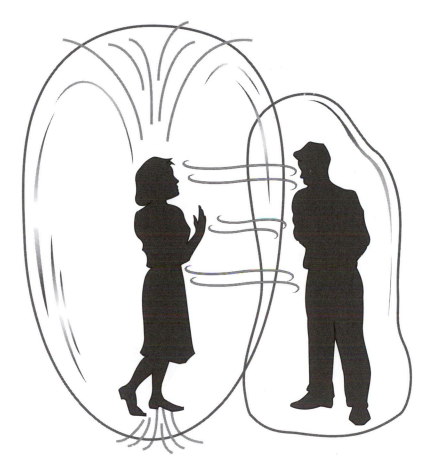

Figure 4.3 Sympathy as a Less Desirable Form of Relating to a Client.

Healer joins client to establish rapport, feels his emotion and distress.

times one person is in need and the other is the nurturer and at other times, the exchange is reversed (see Figure 4.4).

All symbiotic relationships must eventually evolve into more energetically balanced ones to be healthy and positive.

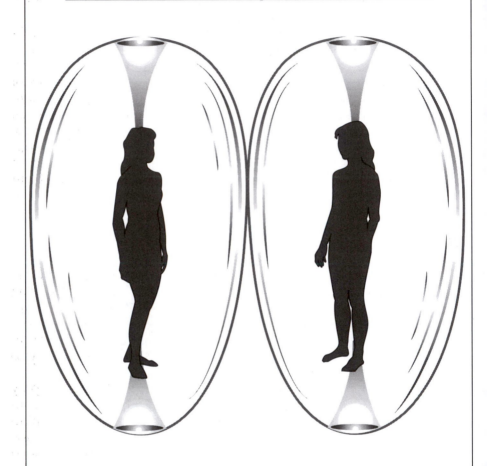

Figure 4.4 Healthy Interactive Relationship Between Friends.

Both fields are full and whole - Synergy - Connecting without overlap.

For example, we might view the symbiosis of parent and baby, the little one totally dependent on the parents for sustenance physically, emotionally, mentally, and spiritually. In other words, in all layers of the energy field. If this were to last a lifetime, it would be pathological, but the evolution in childhood is from dependence to independence, from symbiosis to individual identity. As we mature, we see that interdependence is ultimately the best outcome in the human life cycle, and begin to look for the relationships that allow equal energy exchange or synergy.

Similarly, teacher/student bonds, or therapist/client alliances begin with energetic dependence and evolve to healthy resolution as the client, or student, takes his position as a responsible human being in his own right. Thus, any attempts of teachers to hang on to their students or of therapists to continue therapy indefinitely are energetically unjust. We are all evolving toward greater levels of functioning, and it is appropriate to select teachers and healers on the path of development. At some point, however, we outgrow each teacher or guru and stand in the light of our full creativity to fulfill our human potential.

CENTERING

Centering ourselves as caregivers is the most crucial step in all healing endeavors. Our focused presence before and during any therapeutic interchange creates a strong vibration that appears to lift the client's depleted or distorted field pattern to a higher frequency. Sensing our own central energetic core allows the multiple dimensions of the energy field to come into alignment and harmony.

We also sense that energy flows from the limitless supply in the Universal Field through our focused, intentional consciousness to the client. Centering allows this flow to be unimpeded by our personal issues. To use an analogy, electricity, similar to the flow of energy, is always available, but we need to connect the plug to the wall socket so that the current can be transformed into the correct voltage for turning on a light bulb or machine.

There are literally thousands of ways to center and bring awareness into focus on behalf of the client. It is important for each individual to find the method that works best. For some people, a simple image of a peaceful scene is enough to bring their awareness to a deeper level. Others respond well to working with the breath: one, two, or three strong and long exhales to clear out tension, followed by a smooth and deeper

intake of new air. Some of us connect deeply to music and
can allow ourselves to hear a song or a calming phrase internally. Movement is another powerful way to bring ourselves
into alignment. We can shake out tension in the body and
then add a short dance of moving from side to side or a short
tai ch'i sequence.

It is important to be able to access the state of inner calm
readily. Therefore, practice is essential. We can focus inward
while we are waiting for someone; we can feel all parts of the
body while driving or walking; we can notice how we get
dressed or brush our teeth. Every part of daily life can be
blessed with frequent moments of inner awareness. We can
ask ourselves "How am I feeling right now?" "How could I be
more comfortable?" "What do I need to say or express?"

Before beginning any therapeutic intervention, we want to
make sure we have cleared out as much of our personal agendas as possible. Since none of us is perfect, it is vital that we are
aware of our issues and how we are working with them, lest
any personal distress impede the full flow of energy to the receiver. In addition, a mantra or affirmation of our intent on behalf of the client is helpful. For example, we can focus on a
phrase such as, "I now ask that everything I do at this time be
for my client's highest good." This effectively removes us from
trying to direct the outcome of the intervention because we
truly do not know what is best for our clients from an energetic
perspective. We can trust that the energy will be used by the
client's field in the manner that is most in alignment with her ultimate goals.

Exercise: Centering and Focusing Consciousness

1. Set aside a few moments of quiet before beginning a
counseling session. Release your breath fully several
times to unwind from physical or emotional pressures.

2. Let your inhalations become the "breath of life," bringing in the vitality of the unlimited Universal Energy
Field.

3. Release the old. Bring in the new. As your body responds to the inflow of new energy, sense a flowing
light of warmth and caring moving to every part of
your body, bringing nourishment and wholeness to
any area where there is discomfort or tension.

4. Continuing with the breath as the direct connection to the central core of your energy field, sense each of the layers of your being moving into balance and harmony.

5. Sense the warm glow of your energy field protecting you. Allow yourself to take in as much sunlight and radiant beauty of the Universe as possible. Feel the joy of your aliveness in all parts of your being.

6. As you think of the person you will next encounter, affirm that you can maintain this fullness and joy. Set your intent to be an energy resource for your client's highest good without having to anticipate the outcome of the interaction. Be open to the mystery and magic of the moment; trust your skills and intuition.

7. Gently return to full presence, ready for the interaction.

SUMMARY

We have looked at the multidimensional nature of the human energy field, the specific layers, and the integration of the whole. We have viewed human interactions, including those in psychotherapy, from an energetic perspective. By contrasting sympathy and empathy, we have become aware of the optimal energy field rapport between two persons in dialogue. Setting our intent and focus first allows us as therapists to enter the interaction from a centered state of consciousness.

In the next chapters, we will explore specific ways of using this energetic awareness to assess the energy field and the individual energy centers so that we can move toward increasingly effective therapeutic interventions.

REFERENCES

Brennan, B. *Hands of Light*. New York: Bantam Books, 1987.

Bruyere, R., and Farrens, J. *Wheels of Light*, San Madre, CA: Bon Publishers, 1989, p. 247–259.

Hover-Kramer, D. *Energetic Impressions of Egypt*. Poway, CA: Behavioral Health Consultants, 1993.

Hunt, V. *Infinite Mind: The Science of Human Vibrations*. Malibu, CA: Malibu Publishing Co. 1995.

Kunz, D. *The Personal Aura*. Wheaton, IL: Quest Books, 1991.

Masters, R.S. *The Goddess Sekhmet*. St. Paul, MN: Llewelyn Publications, 1991.

Chapter

5 | THE PSYCHOLOGICAL MEANING OF EACH ENERGY CENTER

In the previous chapter, we discussed the layers of the human energy field and their relation to the dynamic whole. We want to keep in mind that the aura, or field extending beyond the physical body, is only a part of the energetic picture. *Meridians* are energy flow lines that course throughout the human body and form the basis of the science of acupuncture. They have been identified for over five thousand years in the Oriental literature. In addition, there are numerous energy centers, called *chakras* in ancient Sanskrit texts, that we can describe in relationship to the human body and the layers of the energy field. Since these centers of consciousness have particular meaning to physical as well as emotional healing, we will explore them in more depth here.

THE SEVEN MAJOR ENERGY CENTERS

The word *chakra* comes from the Sanskrit meaning *wheel*. Like the ancients, we might picture the energy centers as wheels or vortices of energy, each spinning in its unique way to interconnect the layers of the human energy field. For example, there are energetic vortices at each joint in the human body, apparently generated by the flow of energy, *prana*, or *ch'i* whenever the joint moves. The 206 bones of the human body have many articulations, so we can conclude that there are a great number of these intersections, called the *minor chakras*. These centers are active and vibrant in a well-functioning juncture that has energy flowing freely through it. They are flat or absent in a dysfunctional articulation, such as the immobile, fixed joints seen in severe forms of arthritis.

There are seven major chakras associated with the head and spinal column that provide valuable information about the overall functioning of the individual. These centers have been described in detail by many authors, notably Bailey (1978), Tansley (1985), Rama, et al. (1981), Brennan (1987), and Joy (1979). We encourage the reader to peruse these excellent references as it is not our purpose to detail their many observations. Each of the writers gives a slightly different interpretation to the chakras. We can assume that individual authors come from differing frames of reference and a variety of internal, intuitive experiences. Our purpose here is to present in greater detail the psychological meaning of the chakras, including the interconnecting emotional, mental, and spiritual aspects of each center.

In Figure 5.1 we see the seven major energy centers in relation to the human body as well as to the layers of the energy field. Each energy center interacts with the layers of the field. When the center is open, it allows an inflow of energy from the larger, universal energy field into itself and from there to the various dimensions or layers of the field, bringing moment-by-moment responsiveness and vibrancy to the whole flowing system (see Figure 5.2). For our discussion, it is important to keep this integrative function in mind as each chakra communicates and interacts with all the layers of the field. Thus, when even a single center is cleared through the healer's energetic intervention, it becomes more vibrant, thereby increasing the client's overall sense of vitality and well-being.

The most essential energy flow arises from our connection to the earth and the earth's vital electromagnetic energy field. Rosalyn Bruyere (personal communication, 1993) states that whenever we are disconnected from the earth for any length of time, our energy field becomes gradually depleted. Therefore, what is known as "jet-lag" due to air travel is related to the lessening of our human energy field when we lose contact with the earth. Astronauts exhibit this depletion in

Figure 5.1 Location of the 7 Major Energy Centers

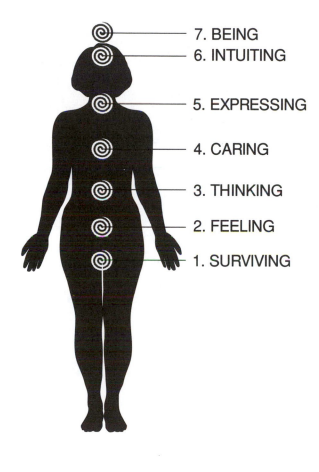

7. BEING
6. INTUITING
5. EXPRESSING
4. CARING
3. THINKING
2. FEELING
1. SURVIVING

more extreme forms; it is well known that their loss of physical vitality is a major hazard of space travel. Nurses especially have been learning about energy field theory to increase their

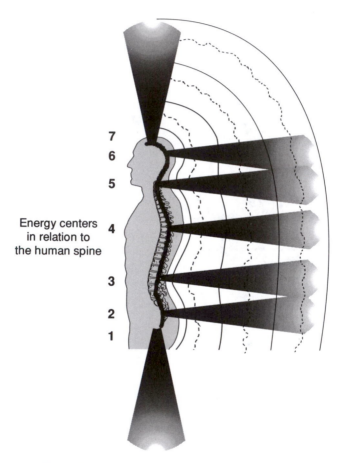

Figure 5.2 Interrelationship of Energy Centers With the Layers of the Field

7
6
5

Energy centers
in relation to
the human spine   4

3

2

1

Expanding vortices of energy through 4 major layers
suggesting psychological impact on whole person

understanding of noninvasive methods for balancing the human energy field. For this reason, Martha Rogers, the distinguished nursing theorist, envisioned that nurses would be in great demand for the future development of space travel (Rogers, 1992).

We can begin our exploration of the energy centers by starting at the base of the spine with the *root* or *base chakra.* If the flow of energy is diminished in the root, the flow to the other centers is impaired. The root chakra is, therefore, the first area of concern in energetic assessment. The second center is in relation to the sacrum and is usually called the *sacral center.* The third is located near the solar plexus of the physical body and is most often called the *solar plexus* or *power center.*

As we move higher, the energy of the centers becomes finer and more subtle. The *heart center,* located in the middle of the chest, is considered by many to be the transformative center. It allows a shift from the gross, more basic energy of the three lower centers to the more ethereal, higher centers. The fifth center is in front of and behind the middle of the neck and is called the *throat chakra.* The *brow center* is sixth and some texts refer to it as the *intuitive center,* or as the "third eye." At the top of the head above the fontanel (the last skull bones to fuse in a baby's head) lies the *crown center.* It relates us to the expanding universe and our sense of connection with a Higher Power. In many texts in the tradition of yoga, three or five more chakras are believed to exist above the crown, completing our magnificent, vibrant structure as energetic beings.

OPTIMUM FUNCTION OF THE MAJOR CENTERS

As we have noted, each chakra is related to the human body and, therefore, has a vital part in optimal physical functioning. The easiest way to conceptualize this is to image each energy center associated with the zone or area of the body to which it is in closest proximity.

The root chakra relates to the hips, legs, feet, and the eliminative functions of the bladder and lower bowels. It is also connected with the body's survival mechanism through the adrenal endocrine glands that trigger our fight/flight response to stress. The sacral center is associated with the lower abdomen, the functions of food and fluid assimilation, and the endocrine reproductive glands. The solar plexus center correlates to the upper abdomen, early digestion of foods and fluids, and is most associated with the pancreatic enzyme insulin that regulates blood sugar levels in the body.

The heart center is connected rather obviously to the heart, lungs, and the circulation of blood. It is also associated with the immune system, lymphatic flows, and the thymus endocrine gland, a major component of immune system functioning. The throat center correlates with the neck, voice, speech, and the thyroid gland. The brow center is related most directly to the facial nerves, eyes, ears, concrete thinking, and the pituitary gland. To complete the picture, the crown center is affiliated with higher, more complex brain functioning and abstract thinking. Its endocrine connection is with the pineal gland, which has been found to regulate our many biorhythms. These constitute our physical responses to the external environment through various patterns, including the commonly known circadian rhythms and cycles with the seasons in nature.

The fact that each energy vortex has a direct physical association with important body organs, intersections of major blood vessels, nerve plexi, and endocrine glands gives us a fascinating opportunity to help the physical body through energetic means. The impact of this understanding for medical and clinical settings is explored extensively in a recent textbook (Hover-Kramer et al., 1996). The psychological meaning of each energy center and ways of utilizing energetic concepts in psychotherapeutic settings, however, are less familiar. We will present insights from our collective thirty years of experience in working with the human energy field as psychotherapists.

The Root Center: Survival Issues and the Will to Live

In its optimal function, the root center is connected to our sense of vitality and aliveness. Nowhere is the interaction between the physical and emotional, the body/mind connection, more evident than in the physiological survival mechanism that can be triggered by a single crisis or thought pattern. The fight/flight response, catalyzed by the adrenal glands that sit atop the kidneys, enables us to have an intense, quick surge of energy for survival in catastrophic times. Through this response, our ancestors were able to make quick escapes from predators or to stand their ground with added strength. Unfortunately, this intrinsic survival mechanism can become a generalized adaptation response in our modern high stress environments (Selye, 1956). A trip to work, for example, repeated five or more times a week, is enough to bring on several episodes of these emergency responses. As every commuter knows, survival on the highways is perilous, and our bodies and emotions carry the daily pressure. Since potentially dangerous situations are often repeated, the body may not fully recover but maintain instead the stress pattern resulting in long-term physical consequences.

Perceived or presumed dangers will trigger the fight/flight response as much as an actual threat to life or limb. Each time we even imagine a dangerous situation, the sympathetic nervous system goes into high gear, repeating stress responses until they become a generalized adaptation. Therefore, we can become more susceptible to many stress-related illnesses, ranging from high blood pressure (essential hypertension) to total systemic collapse. The inability to relax or recover from these high stress responses can also result in immune system illnesses or chronic fatigue immune deficiency syndrome (CFIDS, 1994).

The fact that perceived stress is largely emotional in nature has given us a tremendous opportunity to address physiological problems through mental and emotional processes, such as imagery and relaxation practices. A whole new science of psychoneureoimmunology (Rossi, 1986) has developed in the last decade to address the profound mind/body interconnection.

In the psychological dimension, the root chakra regulates the flow of the vital life force into our bodies, allowing us to feel enthusiastic about life. For many people this flow of vitality is severely limited because of the kinds of distress mentioned. The person may describe herself as being half-alive, or "just hanging on" in a despairing way. Some people are not even certain about wanting to be alive, existing in fear and self-doubt, without joy or enthusiasm.

Jerry was such a client. A series of vague symptoms led him to a number of medical specialists who could not identify any physical problem. Out of frustration he finally sought counseling help. Again, there were only vague symptoms: some depression, a sense of disinterest in others, poor interpersonal relationships, and no sense of life goals or purpose. He was merely going through the motions of functioning normally. Assessment of his energy field showed a completely blocked root chakra with a very small energy field. All of Jerry's affect was gray, vague, and tenuous. When the therapist asked him about his will to live, he gave a blank stare and admitted that he really never wanted to be alive. Since early childhood he felt that his birth was an accident, soon to be corrected by some life-ending disaster. He was literally in limbo.

Obviously there are many therapeutic approaches with a client such as Jerry. An energy-oriented approach would reach to the core issues of his half-hearted life quickly. Attention to the depleted root chakra could help to increase the flow of vitality and give him tools to look at the world in new ways. Affirmations to establish new mental patterns could be "I feel my body," "I feel my life force," "I now enjoy being alive on the earth at this time." This would, of course, be supported by exploration of his feelings and by helping him to explore ways of being more fully alive.

As the flow of energy increases through the root chakra, the other energy centers can also begin to fill with energy and vitality. This mechanism of bringing in the dynamic life force is called the opening of the *kundalini* flow in the yoga tradition (Gopi Krishna, 1988).

The Sacral Center: Opening to Feelings and Choices

The second energy center, the sacral, is empowered by an open root center. The lower abdominal area is one that is often guarded, especially if there has been a history of childhood abuse or sexual invasion. In these instances, the center is blocked as a protective response. The pattern of emotional protectiveness is often evidenced by a form of physical armoring with excess weight in the pelvic area. Emotionally, it is apparent in persons who isolate themselves and have difficulty knowing or expressing their feelings. Because it is too painful to bring up feelings associated with the past, more positive emotions in the present cannot be fully enjoyed.

There are understandably many distortions when this energy center is blocked. On the one hand, we may see a person who has difficulty in intimate relationships for fear of connecting with pain. This is the client to whom it just seems easier to avoid human contact. On the other hand, we may see a person who chooses some addictive, compulsive means of feeling closer to others. The addictive patterns may be related to a chemical dependence, such as drugs, alcohol, nicotine, caffeine, or sugars. Alternately, there can be behavioral addiction, such as hysteria, sexual addiction, or co-dependency, including loyalty to others far beyond logical reason. The issues are akin to the physiological functions of the chakra, the assimilation and elimination of fluids and foods. Psychologically this translates into selecting appropriate relationships, assimilating ideas from others, and being able to release what is not needed or useful.

Work with the sacral center, then, would first address permission to access feelings. This involves full expression of the feelings around past events as well as being more aware of one's current emotions. Often, when therapists move the hands over the lower abdominal center, a flood of memories will emerge spontaneously. Reconnecting with forgotten, repressed material can bring great relief, or catharsis. It is also our experience that some clients will simply release blocked material in a large energetic mass without specific cognitive detail. This is especially true when the repressed material is related to a childhood event that occurred before verbal and cognitive processes were fully established.

The Solar Plexus Center: Thinking, Control, and Power

The third chakra is the center most related to power issues. In the physical body, the solar plexus is a great intersection of major blood vessels, nerve ganglia, and essential body organs. In the energy field, the solar plexus region is the storage battery, the repository of extra energy for lean times. Our sense of personality or ego identity and power is most supported by this center. Clear thinking, decision-making, and figuring out solutions to problems—in short, the signs of effective ego-functioning—are associated with this center. Assertive and effective communication with others is another hallmark of healthy aspects of the solar plexus chakra.

 Distortions in the energy flow of this center can result in being overly controlling or excessively passive. Because it is virtually impossible to be totally inert, a very passive person may explode when his limits are exceeded. This sudden explosiveness may seem overwhelming and aggressive to others because it comes out of the frustration of unclear boundaries. Clinically, this dynamic is termed *passive-aggressive behavior* and creates a great deal of confusion, both in the person and in his social environment.

On the other hand, controlling every part of our lives and other people is equally impossible. Manipulating others is usually not appreciated and takes a tremendous toll on the quality of relationships.

We note, for example, a successful businessman like Pete, who excelled in his career by being compulsive and detail-oriented. At home Pete acted like a virtual tyrant, and his behavior was destroying family life. His children demonstrated poor self-esteem and underdeveloped personalities because much of their early lives was dictated by the absolute control of their father. Pete's wife became withdrawn and increasingly incommunicative as Pete tried to run his household "like a tight ship." The sexual acting out behavior of their oldest daughter finally brought the family into counseling where some resolution became possible.

The lower three energy centers are connected to major psychological functions: a sense of vitality, the willingness to express and connect with feelings, and the ability to think and communicate assertively. In our experience, over 90% of all psychotherapeutic issues relate to dysfunction of the lower three centers. We will explore specific emotional conditions and relevant energetic approaches later in this book, but first we will continue to look at the emotional meaning of the upper, more subtle energy centers.

The Heart Center: Unconditional Caring and Forgiveness

The heart-centered emotion is one of unconditional caring and forgiveness. This stands in contrast to possessive, security-seeking, or needy love and is characterized by the attachments made through the lower centers. When the energy of the heart center is open and flowing, we find that our capacity for accepting others, just as they are, expands. Even though we may see another's faults, we do not hold onto grudges but rather forgive readily. Furthermore, with open heart centers, we can accept ourselves, including our shadow aspects, and obvious faults. Things literally begin to lighten up as we open our hearts energetically. Humor, and being able to step back from over-involvement with others, is possible from this perspective.

For many people, the heart center never really has an opportunity to develop. This would be characteristic of the person who is caught up in lukewarm commitments, lack of emotional depth, or a poor sense of personal identity. We appropriately speak of such a person as being "half-hearted."

Obviously, the support of the lower centers is needed to move us into a genuine sense of positive regard toward self and others. The depth of caring for others can only emerge out of the fullness of an open heart center. Though many caregivers may not recognize this, it is literally not possible to love others without healthy self-esteem.

It is also possible for religious fervor to cloud the heart-centered functions. Although the Scriptures clearly say, "Thou shalt love others as your self," self-respect and self-nurturing are not often taught in traditional religions. For example, some clients report incredible injustices in their childhood years while attending parochial schools. Jim, a young adult client, recalled being beaten by the teaching nuns because he liked to keep allowance money in his pocket. In the name of their "love" they told him he was selfish and ridiculed him in front of the class. Feeling shamed and defeated, he later had difficulty being successful in many aspects of his adult life. In spite of their choosing a caregiving profession, the teachers demonstrated little love for themselves or the children entrusted to their care.

The Throat Center: Creativity and Expression

Out of a deepening sense of self-esteem, and with the support of the full heart center, a tremendous outflow of creative self-expression can become available. The throat chakra empowers the joy of being ourselves that can be expressed in many ways. Almost any activity has within it the potential for creativity. It can be as simple as making a small place of beauty in one's home, writing a poem, singing a song, or sharing an idea. The quickest way to transform energy is to tap into the beauty of nature through a picture, a memory, or even a single blade of grass. Through these simple practices we are reminded that there is virtually no limit to the creative potential of any given moment.

Blockage of energy in the throat center is characterized by withholding one's creative impulses. Unfortunately, many of us interpreted childhood instructions to be quiet to mean holding back. Healing of this center is related to speaking out, expressing one's self, and one's sense of truth clearly. As clients heal the distortions of the lower centers, creativity becomes the essential next step in evolution. This goal is supported by working with the intuitive potentials.

The Brow Center: Seeing with Intuition and Compassion

The intuitive center is the brow chakra. As psychological strengths develop, the ability to see with insight follows. With the support of the lower centers, we are able to look at others with compassion and true empathy. Along with this response comes an intuitive grasp of another person's situation. Often, as sensitivity develops, we are able to sense a whole sequence of events that led up to the present situation or to actually see the images that occurred in someone's life. This is really not so unusual as we might think. Intuition is simply the ability to see, hear, or sense with our higher perceptive capacities. It involves an attunement to all of our perceptions through the physical senses and seems to be one of our birthrights as evolving, healthy human beings.

Constriction of the brow energy center would, of course, impair this flow of insight or possibly cause us to be critical of others, thinking we are incapable of understanding their dilemmas. Another serious distortion of this center is the desire for an intuitive grasp without taking on the strenuous work of mastering the lower centers. The wish to transcend and to become intuitive quickly has been the impetus of many ill-fated drug trips. The result, unfortunately, can be the energetic equivalent of running a 220-volt current through wiring that only has a 10-volt capacity. In other words, the individual literally burns out nerve pathways through impatience, and may suffer lifelong physical and emotional damage as a result.

Our discussion suggests that intuition can and does develop naturally as we mature. However, there are no shortcuts, no spiritual bypasses or quick fixes. Superficial attempts to adopt someone else's path of intuition, such as obtaining a psychic reading or following a guru, are usually not effective in the long run. The path to intuition has to develop in its unique way, one that fits each unique individual.

The Crown Center: Connecting to the Transpersonal

The open and flowing crown center puts us in touch with dimensions that are greater than our personal selves and is often called the *transpersonal realm.* For some, this may be a sense of connecting to a personal Higher Power whereas for others it simply may be feeling at peace with nature or the universe.

Expression of this dimension is highly individualistic, because each person has a special way of expressing spiritual truth. No matter how we choose to speak of this quality, there is a joyfulness and peacefulness when the crown is open. We catch a glimpse that there is cohesiveness and unity around us and the world begins to make sense.

Technically, there are no distortions in the crown since we are always connected to our Source or unifying principle. However, we can easily limit our thinking, including our beliefs about the Infinite. It is as if we choose to be obsessed with our limitations, such as with the clouds of a rainy day, instead of remembering that the sun is always present. Reconnecting by means of centering (described in Chapter 4) is an energetic intervention to help maintain the flow of energy from the root through the crown chakras.

VIBRATIONAL PATTERNS OF THE ENERGY CENTERS

Each center of consciousness emits a distinctive vibrational pattern that nurtures the entire human energy system. The unique vibrations of the chakras, from simple to increasingly complex spins, have been extensively documented by intuitive healers throughout the ages, notably Dr. Charles Leadbeater in the West (1927). Detailed research confirms that the wave emissions from a meditator, who is focusing attention on a specific energy center, yield a frequency that corresponds to the colors that have been reported by clairvoyant persons (Hunt, 1995). The colors that correspond to each of the energy centers are, as one might intuit, the colors of the rainbow, beginning with the slower frequency of red and moving to the very rapid vibrations of indigo, purple, and lavender.

Sound, as another dimension of the electromagnetic spectrum, also registers the various vibrational frequencies of the chakras. Throughout recorded history, specific tonal patterns have been used to enhance the human sense of well-being and harmony. The sequence of tones known as a scale in music (do-re-mi-fa-sol-la-ti-do) corresponds to the chakra vibration patterns. Among other current writers about the power of sound in healing, Ted Andrews compiled a study of tones and vowels used cross-culturally to enhance function of the energy centers in *Sacred Sounds* (1993).

To bring the various aspects of the vibrational nature of the energy centers into focus, we include the following chart as a reference (see Table 5.1).

Another way of approaching the understanding of the energy centers is by incorporating them into a meditative practice. The following sequence suggests a way the counselor could voice-guide a client to increase self-awareness by focusing on the distinctive centers of consciousness.

TABLE 5.1

Energy Center	Physical Areas of Influence	Major Psychological Function	Color	Sound
Root	Feet, legs, thighs, hips, perineal floor	***Connecting*** to survival, safety, security, sense of vitality, joy in being alive	Red	"do" C on piano
Sacral	Lower abdomen, pelvis, assimilation and release	***Feeling*** letting emotions serve as sensors, choosing and releasing	Orange	"re" D
Solar Plexus	Upper abdomen, early digestion	***Thinking*** sense of power, identity, control, self-esteem, effective assertion	Yellow	"mi" E
Heart	Chest, heart, blood and lymphatic flows	***Caring*** positive accepting of self and others, unconditional forgiveness	Green	"fa" F
Throat	Throat and neck	***Expressing*** creative self-awareness, playfulness, humor, singing, writing, etc.	Light Blue	"sol" G
Brow	Face, eyes, ears, lower cerebral function	***Seeing*** clearly, clairvoyance, insight, compassion	Indigo Blue	"la" A
Crown	Upper brain, biorhythms	***Being*** connecting to spirit, alignment with Higher Will, fullfilling one's sense of purpose and meaning	Purple, Lavender White	"ti" and "do" B, and C (in higher octave)

Exercise: Chakra Meditation Sequence

1. Make sure you are comfortable. Relax and exhale fully, releasing tension from the body and mind.

2. Allow your awareness to rest at the base of the spine. Sense the flow of the color red moving from the base of the spine to fill your entire body with a sense of aliveness and vitality.

3. Focus your inner awareness with the breath and allow your attention to move to the lower abdomen. Feel the color orange filling the area with warmth and let your whole body sense the permission to feel all of the emotions. Note the ones that are comfortable and the ones that are not.

4. Let your attention move to the upper abdomen, the color yellow, and permission to think clearly. Sense your whole being filled with a sense of power to effectively take charge of your life and relationships.

5. Sense your focus at the heart center. Image the color green, perhaps as a deep forest green, filling your whole being with a sense of unconditional acceptance. Extend your caring to your loved ones and allow yourself to receive their caring in the heart area.

6. Move awareness to the throat area with the color of sky blue or turquoise. Feel your creativity expand; notice the things you have made that give you joy and commit to a specific creative activity for the next week.

7. Let your consciousness shift to the brow area. Connect with your compassion and intuition. Let the color of indigo blue support your ability to see and hear.

8. Sense the area above your crown and the connection with All That Is, the divine plan in your life. The colors of purple, and lighter shades of lavender, white, and silver enhance the expanding consciousness of your being, whole and alive.

9. Gently bring your awareness to your feet and hands, feeling the breath as the connecting link between all the steps. Set your focus and intent for your next task, feeling the support of a friendly universe.

SUMMARY

We have looked at the major human energy centers with special focus on the psychological aspects. Because the psyche and soma are so closely interrelated, issues will often surface in the emotional dimension of the field before manifesting in the denser, physical body. Predictable life crises, such as the loss of a loved one, can cause significant shifts in the organization of the human energy field. As grief reactions considerably diminish the field, it is helpful to work with them early before the pattern of decreased energy flow affects the weakest aspect of the physical dimension with resulting illness.

Working with the human energy field for emotional issues thus provides a useful resource for preventing physical breakdown. In addition, we can work directly with each of the energy centers to assist with psychological concerns such as self-esteem, awareness of feelings, and effective self-expression, as we shall discuss in later chapters.

REFERENCES

Andrews, T. *Sacred Sounds*. St. Paul, MN: Llewellyn Publications, 1993.

Bailey, A. *Esoteric Healing*. London: Lucis Publishing Co., 1978.

Brennan, B. *Hands of Light*. New York: Bantam Books, 1987.

Hunt, V. *Infinite Mind: The Science of Human Vibrations*. Malibu, CA: Malibu Publishing Co., 1995.

Joy, B. *Joy's Way*. Los Angeles: J.P. Tarcher, Inc., 1979.

Krishna, G. (Kieffer, G., ed.) *Kundalini for the New Age*. New York: Bantam Books, 1988.

Leadbeater, C. *The Chakras*. Wheaton, IL: Theosophical Publishing House, 1927.

Rama, S., Ballentine, R., and Ayjaya, S. *Yoga and Psychotherapy*. Honesdale, PA: Himalayan International Institute, 1981.

Rogers, M. "Nursing science and the space age." *Nursing Science Quarterly*, 5:1, 1992, p. 27–34.

Rossi, E.L. *The Psychobiology of Mind-Body Healing*. New York: W.W. Norton, 1986.

Selye, H. *The Stress of Life*. New York: McGraw-Hill, 1956.

———, "A Guide to CFIDS." *CFIDS Chronicle*. Winter, 1994.

Tansley, D.V. *Subtle Body*. New York: Thames and Hudson, Inc., 1985.

6

ASSESSMENT OF THE HUMAN ENERGY FIELD

As we have suggested, working with the human energy field can be a valuable adjunct in dealing with emotional issues. In addition to the interconnection with body physiology, each chakra has specific psychological meanings that influence the entire human energy system.

We might picture this human energy system as a dynamic, evolving, ever-changing configuration. The patterns are interwoven like the threads of a tapestry, although at times distinctive layers of the field are apparent. Like the many colors within an iridescent opal, all layers are interconnected with each other. The individual's current state of consciousness determines which dimension predominates at a given time. For example, if a strong emotion such as anger is present, the color red will most likely be apparent, emanating from the root energy center and the emotional layer of the field. If the individual is calm and thoughtful, a smooth band of yellow may be most evident, suggesting activation of the mental layer and the related third chakra.

As therapists and counselors, we want to keep in mind two major areas of concern when assessing the human energy field for emotional issues. The first is related to the overall pattern in the field. This can be sensed by making slow sweeps with the hands from head to toe several inches away from the client's body. In doing so, we notice whether the field is symmetrical and full, or distorted in some way. Asymmetry between the two sides suggests an energetic imbalance. Similarly, over-expansion of one half of the torso compared to the other tells us that there is a distortion of some kind. This can occur with the upper or lower torso, or with the right and left sides. At times, we will notice constrictions in the field, which feel like blocks or irregularities over an affected part of the body or in the emotional field.

By setting our intent for assessing individual layers, we can intuitively sense the edges of each layer. For example, as the healer sets his centered intention and focus for assessing the emotional layer, he will be able to access the emotional dimension of the field. Because this layer is less structured than the etheric or mental layers (described in Chapter 4), he will notice the soft, almost fluffy, irregular shape of the emotional dimension. Distortions in the emotional field in relation to the client's individual chakras can also be noted with this assessment. In a similar fashion, the mental layer can be accessed, giving information about the overall pattern of this dimension as well as the mental aspect of each of the energy centers.

The other consideration for assessment is the specific condition of each of the major energy centers. Since the chakras are directly associated with such core issues as the will to live, the ability to feel, and the sense of identity, power and control, we can receive much valuable feedback from determining the condition of each center. The individual chakras in the etheric field can be felt by placing one's hands 1–4 inches above their physical location as described in Chapter 5. Assessment of the condition of the energy centers in other layers can occur as the healer sets his intent.

We now explore these two assessment considerations in more detail.

THE EFFECT OF BLOCKED ENERGY CENTERS

As we have described, the flow of energy, *prana*, or *ch'i* in the human energy system is dynamic and multidimensional. The human energy system encompasses the layers of the field extending beyond and through the physical body, the meridians and acupressure points, and the energy centers. Like a beautiful river, energy flows from its source, the limitless supply of energy in the Universal Energy Field, into the chakras and to all the related dimensions of the field.

Nurtured from this input, energy flows out to the external world through our creativity, self-expression, and actions. If this river is blocked for any reason, the energy flow is diminished. Over time, this leads to stillness and pooling in the areas above the constriction, and depletion due to insufficient energy flow in the areas below the impediment. Like a stagnant river, the energetic body no longer receives sufficient nourishment for productivity. This results in blocked flow of creativity and, ultimately, limited capacity to enjoy the fullness of life.

The analogy of a river that has a constriction of its flow pattern, with resulting impoverished life on its banks, is very apt when we think of the blockage created by emotional trauma. Consider, for example, the impact of abandonment by an intimate friend. Initially, there may be a sense of shock or desire to forget the whole experience. Over time, however, the client's response patterns can become hardened, creating emotional barriers or obstructions to new relationships. The sufferer may attempt to deny the feeling of loss and suppress the hurtful event. This pattern of emotional armoring becomes more pervasive as the client builds barriers to new relationships in order to protect herself against further possibilities of being hurt. In this case, we would consider such an emotional constriction a detriment to the personality structure as it prevents future possibility of healthy, intimate relationships.

Catharsis, or emotional release work, is needed to remove the blocked material. As we will explore in the next chapter, the process of unburdening begins by bringing the energetically contained material to mind, expressing the associated feelings, and moving beyond the old attachment to new insights. The effects of this kind of psychological working through, with the additional resource of energy healing, can be dramatic, quite similar to the effects seen when we remove obstructions from a dammed-up stream of water. The initial response can be a huge swell of emotion, appropriately called "*flooding*," followed by gradual balancing of the emotions leading to a more peaceful, harmonious inner landscape.

Each chakra, with its unique qualities as a center of consciousness, communicates energetically to the whole system. Through the energy centers we gain information about the effects of emotional distortion and the resulting impact on the energy flow pattern. For example, let us consider the value placed in our culture on high achievement as a manifestation of success. In examining a person like Bill who was highly successful in the business world, the therapist noticed an overactive third chakra with blocked, stagnant energy in the higher centers. He deducted from this that Bill overemphasized his work life, accepting the cultural norm of focusing on financial and job security, to the detriment of his intuitive or self-expressive centers. Areas relating to insight and compassion in the brow center, to creativity in the throat, and to loving acceptance in the heart were unable to receive nurturing flow from the Universal Source. In Bill's case, this energetic distortion resulted in ever-increasing disconnection from the more human, playful, and creative parts of himself. Though outwardly successful, Bill suffered from a sense of alienation, personal insecurity, and emptiness as his professional life soared. Awareness of this sense of inner emptiness is more apparent as persons reach the middle years of forty and fifty, and is often popularly called a "mid-life crisis." In the language of transpersonal psychology, we call this the loss of soul, while more traditional psychological assessment identifies the malaise as depression or loss of libido.

We explore now the many ways that healers can increase their sense of intuitive awareness so that the most effective energetic interventions can be selected in the transformational process.

HIGHER SENSE PERCEPTION OF THE FIELD AND THE CHAKRAS

Students of energetic modalities develop their intuitive skills by working with enhanced sensory perception. All of the senses—seeing, hearing, touching, tasting and smelling—can serve as entry points to awareness of subtler energies. This heightened awareness of energetic frequencies beyond our usual physical perceptions is called *higher sense perception* (*HSP*) by several authors (Brennan, 1987; Karagulla and Kunz, 1989).

Most students of the intuitive start with the sensory data that is personally most comfortable to begin their explorations, and then gradually expand from there to include the other senses. There is truly no best way to begin. We encourage the reader to start with his or her most comfortable sensory mode and then allow the perception of subtle energies to develop along with intuition. We now describe some specific ways to enhance intuitive awareness through each of the senses.

Visual Perception

Throughout recorded time, sensitive people have reported "seeing" beyond ordinary vision. The eye represents one of many ways to access information about subtle energies. Visual cues around the human energy field may vary significantly. In developing these skills, we might first begin to note the difference between light and dark while gently gazing at the space around a client's head or shoulders. Alternately, we may notice an area near the client where the air seems disturbed or turbulent, similar to the colorless exhaust from an engine, the intake area around a moving airline jet, or the wavy heat radiation lines above a hot pavement.

As visual acuity increases with practice, you may be able to note flashes of color around a client. For instance, the color orange may suddenly flash in front of you when you are talking with someone who is very emotional. Or you may note a gray area in relation to a depleted chakra in someone who is depressed. It is helpful to remember that color is most likely to be seen when the person is actually producing a strong emotion. It is much more difficult to sense the colors of someone who is emotionally defended or disconnected.

Another possibility is that of actually seeing shapes around a client. These shapes may be very abstract and diffuse, such as a ball of light, or they may actually resemble a physical object or person. Dora Kunz, for example, described her visual perceptions of the aura using lifelong skills as a clairvoyant in her book, *The Personal Aura* (1991). She was able to discern objects that had become energetically imbedded in her clients' energy fields. When she described what she saw, some clients were able to access specific memory of an emotionally charged situation that had long been forgotten or repressed.

A psychologist friend named Jane recently saw a client who was suffering from undiagnosed abdominal pain at the request of the attending physician. Jane sensed a twisted mass above the abdomen when she looked at the client's energy field. As it turned out, the constriction related to the client's early childhood problems that began with the arrival of a new baby in the family. When the client uncovered her unthinkable wish to choke or twist off the new baby brother's head, she was able to express and release her murderous rage. She began to find relief from her intense pain.

Visual higher sense perception is only one of many pathways that help us to sense subtle energies. Often, visual sensitivity, called *clairvoyance*, emerges spontaneously as the healer continues his practice. In our classes we discourage learners from demanding too much of themselves, such as "seeing" auras or colors associated with the functioning of the energy centers. It seems, in fact, that the more one demands to "see" for assessment purposes, the less likely one is to succeed. However, we want to offer a few suggestions as beginning exercises that may assist the reader in developing visual acuity.

Exercise: Holding a Focus

1. Allow yourself to watch someone who is excitedly talking about his favorite subject. Make sure the background is a single color wall without unusual shadows or lighting. Let your eyes focus on the midline of the talker's face, i.e., the middle of the forehead, nose, mouth, and chin area. Maintaining this focus, let your peripheral vision drift to the right shoulder and neck area, to the left shoulder and neck, and above the head.

2. Notice any movement that you see beyond the physical body, perhaps a color or dark area that seems to emanate and move in little puffs away from the person. Many people are surprised to find how easy this is to do and how much movement there is in the human energy field.

Exercise: Spreading the Fingers

1. Against a dark background with no shadows or unusual lighting, hold the fingers of both hands together so that the tips of the fingers touch.

2. While focusing the eyes on the middle where the fingers meet, gently pull the fingers apart. As you separate the fingers, you may begin to notice white "streamers" of energy and little bulges around each of the fingertips.

Exercise: "Seeing" with a Partner

1. Select a partner who is willing to explore with you. Ask the partner to think of a recent event that evoked a strong emotion. Then ask her to step into the intensity of the feeling for a short time.

2. As your partner does this, allow yourself to imagine a color that might be emitted. Ask your partner which energy center felt most turbulent and note if the color of the activated energy center matches your perception. Try this several times with different emotions, and then exchange the process to let the partner learn as well.

Exercise: Sharing an Image

1. With a partner who is willing, agree on a specific time for sending an image. While you sit quietly and in a centered state, the partner goes outside and selects an object to hold in his hand. At the appointed time, he focuses intently on the image for one minute, sending the image telepathically to you.

2. Record or draw a picture of what you receive at the appointed time. Later, compare experiences and do several exchanges. Remember, everything becomes easier with practice.

Visual perceptions include a wide variety of finer categories, called *submodalities* (Bandler, 1985). Contrast between light and dark is one such category, occurring when we let ourselves notice varying degrees of brightness around a living thing. Other examples include actual perception of movement, air turbulence, or flow of energy. Perception of color and subtle shadings becomes more evident as we pay attention whenever there is a strong emotion expressed by clients. The astute therapist may sense the presence of images from the client's life, especially if the client is recalling a highly significant experience. Additionally, we may be able to sense the presence of someone closely associated with the client. Some clients believe in angels, or other forms of guidance, that assist them in difficult times. This phenomenon accounts for the current flood of best-selling books about angels. Healers who work on subtle energy levels often have a strong sense of the presence of helpful guides who join in the healing process.

Kinesthetic Perception

While over 80% of the general population is predominantly visual, a very high percentage of helping professionals are predominantly kinesthetic, that is, most comfortable with the sense of touch. Their perception of subtle energies begins through the sense of touch, and they can most readily describe what they feel with their hands.

The skin is the primary sensory organ from birth, long before our other senses develop. Neurophysiologists also tell us that from the moment of early neurological development in the embryonic stage, we respond to our environment kinesthetically. Understandably, the sense of touch is the most highly complex of all the senses and affords a seemingly endless variety of submodalities.

Consider for a moment the many things we can sense with our hands: temperature differences; textures of cloth or objects; tension on top of the skin; tension underneath the skin; muscular tension; pressure ranging from a feather-light touch to the massive weight of a boulder; pain, ranging from an exquisite tickle to itching, burning, throbbing, and bone-aching discomfort; degrees of wetness and dryness in the air; electrical charges or vibrations; the slightest nuance of air movement to gale force winds; and even the sense of someone's presence or absence in a large room.

Blind persons rely on this kinesthetic diversity to move around without bumping into things and to "read" in Braille. In fact, some blind persons have learned to differentiate color with their hands. These people are valuable in certain work situations, such as in the detection of color-coded wires in underground telephone conduits.

It is no wonder that the sense of touch is most associated with energy-oriented healing. It lends its name to well-known modalities of this work, such as Therapeutic Touch and Healing Touch. Apparently, touch readily connects us to our intuitive awareness of the human energy field. An interesting study was done by Therapeutic Touch practitioner Nancy France in which a sample of eleven children, all under ten years of age, were taught to sense the energy field around one of their friends. All of the children reported some spontaneous sensation of touch, describing their experiences as "tingly," "like static," and "like a vacuum cleaner when I'm bringing up dust" (France, 1993, p. 36).

Exercise: Sensing with the Hands

1. Because each of us is an energy field, we can initially begin practicing kinesthetic awareness by working with our own hands and our own fields. Try gently passing the hands over the face about six inches away and notice how that feels to your hands. Note also how it feels to the face.

2. Next, pass the hands over a part of the body where there is discomfort or tension. Does it feel fuller or less vibrant than the face? Is it warmer or cooler? Is there tingling or vibration? If you wish, compare a painful area with a part of the body that feels strong or with one of the major energy centers.

Exercise: Developing Sense of Touch with a Partner

1. Sit across from a friend who is willing and allow a moment to center. Feel the flow of energy through your body, in your chest, and in your arms and hands. Let your hands face the partner's hands, palm to palm, and notice how far apart you can move the palms and still feel some fullness or flow between you.

2. Try pointing a finger into your partner's palm, an inch or so away, and notice the sensation of the more focused energy pattern. Draw a design in your partner's palm and have your partner describe the outline of the design. Next, draw a pattern several inches away from the skin. How does your partner know what you are doing? What words describe the experience? Maybe, like the children mentioned above, you can invent your own words to describe the sensations, such as "fluffy," "fuzzy," "bouncy," "vibrating," or "magnetic."

Auditory Perception

While only a small portion of the general population uses the auditory sense as the primary means of sensory input, sound is a powerful influence on the human psyche. For the millennia before written communication, the aural mode was the primary method for carrying information from one generation to the next. Storytelling and singing are two innate human capacities. They serve as valuable, primary communication tools with children and in primitive cultures even today.

Through our sense of hearing we can determine emotional meaning even when only a single word is used. Consider, for example, the word "really" and hear it in various intonations that give it totally different meanings. These might be praise, criticism, or special emphasis, perceived through mere changes in the speaker's voice tone. Skilled therapists are attuned to such inflections in their clients' voices that reveal underlying feelings often outside the person's awareness.

There are a wide variety of submodalities within the sense of hearing as well. We have tone and pitch that can completely change meanings of a word, as in tonal languages such as Chinese. The quality of a sound may vary greatly in timbre, which is the vibrational pattern of the sound waves produced. Differences in timbre enable us to differentiate between instruments of an orchestra even though they may all play the same note, as the "A" with which they tune. Further, melody is decidedly different in structure from chords, and harmony is dramatically distinct from dissonance. Rhythms are basic to the human body. The heartbeat can be felt as well as heard by most of us when we are truly quiet. And we can note the contrast between a pleasing, regular beat and an irritating, syncopated one.

As higher sense perception develops, some sensitives become clairaudient, perceiving information through subtle sounds. They may "hear" irregular rhythms, or disharmony, perhaps perceived as a squeak in a disturbed area of the human energy field. In time, the clairaudient person may actually begin to perceive verbal information, "hearing" instructions for healing, or messages that may be helpful to the client.

The Sense of Taste and Smell

Curiously, the senses of taste and smell may also be activated when we work with the human energy field. We might remember that when energy flow is blocked, the pattern remains embedded and stored in the human energy field. In fact, there seems to be good evidence that there is cellular as well as emotional memory of traumatic events, even for those long forgotten by the individual.

Clients who have had surgery may spontaneously release the smell of anesthesia when a healer works in the emotional layer of the energy field. Alternately, people who have long ago stopped smoking may suddenly smell and taste stale to-bacco smoke as they are working through emotional issues. A dramatic example occurred in a classroom with 60 people, all of whom smelled burning rubber during an energy healing demonstration. After checking to ensure that there were no possible fire hazards, we asked one client what had happened to her. Tearfully, she described being in a car accident a year ago in which her shoulder was crushed. The smell of a burn-ing tire was her last memory before losing consciousness. As the teacher moved her hands to clear the shoulder area, the stored trauma, along with its noxious odor, again surfaced.

DOCUMENTATION OF ASSESSMENT

Using the various sensory cues and submodalities we have dis-cussed, we can assess the client's energy field. A hand scan of the client's overall field pattern gives us an idea of where there may be asymmetry suggesting a blocked or overactive area. More detailed assessment over each of the seven major chakras gives us specific information about psychological issues. A healthy, flowing chakra will feel full, vibrant, and show a clock-wise spin on assessment with a pendulum (Brennan, 1987, p. 81), or parallel alignment with two rods (Laskow, 1992, p.142). As the hands move over the chakra area, there will be a sense of something brushing gently against the hands like a feather.

It is useful to develop easy, quick ways of documenting these patterns as a basis for the planning of energetic interven-tions and later evaluation. The chakras are sometimes com-pletely closed, as demonstrated by absence of tingling or vibrancy, stillness, or coolness. In these instances, a symbol, such as a dot (.) can be used. In contrast, various degrees of openness can be indicated by sketching in back and forth movements, elliptical shapes or circles of varying sizes. In a balanced, symmetrical field the chakras are "blended," all ap-proximately equal in size.

Notation of the overall pattern of the field can be made by simply drawing the outline of the pattern around a diagram of the body (see Figures 6.1 and 6.2). The condition of each energy center can be noted as well. Unusual features of indi-vidual layers assessed through the therapist's intuitive ques-tioning can be drawn in. Jotting down different shapes or colors sensed intuitively also provides helpful information. As

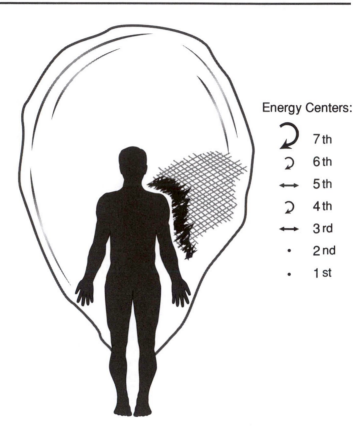

Figure 6.1 Energy Field of a Client with AIDS

Energy Centers:

- 7 th
- 6 th
- 5 th
- 4 th
- 3 rd
- 2 nd
- 1 st

Field Configuration:

Expanded at crown area, dark at left shoulder.
Symptom:
Kaposi's sarcoma
No field palpable at waist or below.
Symptoms:
Depression and neuropathy of feet.

Energy Centers:

1st & 2nd energy centers
closed, no movement.
Upper 4 centers open
to varying degrees,
with crown center
very expanded.

Figure 6.2 Energy Field of a Self Centered Client

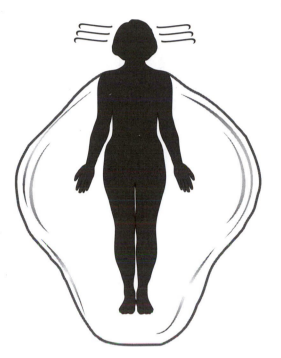

Energy Centers:

- 7 th
- 6 th
← 5 th
← 4 th
↻ 3 rd
↻ 2 nd
← 1 st

Field Configuration:

Tightness around the head with dark bands
Symptom:
Frequent headaches
Over expansion at midd!e, overt sexuality
and addiction to money.
Symptoms:
Difficulty relating to others, lack of insight,
discord at work and in marriage.

Energy Centers:

No movement at crown
or brow centers.
Minimal movement at
throat and heart.
Overdeveloped in 2nd and
3rd energy centers.

the client changes over time, these notations are a valuable aid in noting progress.

One example of energetic pattern notation is of a client who has AIDS, illustrated in Figure 6.1. We see the overall depletion of the energy field with a burst of energy at the head, suggesting that the intuitive and spiritual resources are developing as the client faces his life-threatening illness. The root and second chakras are totally blocked in association with the lack of physical vitality. There is slight movement over the solar plexus, heart, and throat centers. Intuitive assessment of the emotional field shows blockage in the root center related to fear or anger, and a diminished throat center suggests that strong emotions are being held back rather than expressed.

The second illustration presents the energetic pattern of a client presenting with emotional hyperactivity, symptoms of phobia, emotional lability, and hysteria (Figure 6.2). Here we see a field configuration that shows preoccupation with the lower parts of the body, sexuality, and the related energy centers. The upper centers are almost totally blocked, suggesting that the client has great difficulty putting herself in someone else's place or connecting with a sense of higher purpose in her life. Her energy pattern suggests she is overly focused on bodily sensations while lacking a sense of inner strength and connection with her intuitive dimensions.

SUMMARY

We have now sharpened our basic tools for assessment of the human energy field. Starting with the most comfortable sensory mode, we develop awareness of the various submodalities and fine-tune our higher sense perceptions. Gradually, subtle cues from the other senses blend in to provide a quick, intuitive grasp of the client's affective domain.

As therapists, we begin by asking the client's permission to scan the field. We assess the field as a whole to sense the overall configuration, followed by attention to the nature of individual energy centers and layers. We then record the results of assessment on the psychoenergetic intake sheet (see sample in Appendix B). Over time, we may find repeated patterns of blockage in a specific client's field, and begin to notice energetic configurations associated with certain disorders. The energetic assessment builds the foundation for development of the psychoenergetic healing process that we will explore in the next section.

REFERENCES

Bandler, R. *Using Your Brain for a Change*. Moab, UT: Real People Press, 1985, p. 21–26.

Brennan, B. *Hands of Light*. New York: Bantam Books, 1987.

France, N.E.M. "The child's perception of the human energy field using therapeutic touch." *Journal of Holistic Nursing* 11:2, 1993.

Karagulla, S., & Kunz, D. *The Chakras and the Human Energy Field*. Wheaton, IL: Theosophical Publishing House, 1989.

Kunz, D. *The Personal Aura*. Wheaton IL: Quest Books, 1991.

Laskow, L. *Healing with Love*. San Francisco, CA: HarperCollins Publishers, 1992.

III | CONCEPTS OF ENERGY HEALING

In this section, we consider the actual steps of the psychoenergetic healing intervention. This is followed by an understanding of imagery as an interactive part of healing work in the psychoenergetic sequence. Then, the self-transcending awareness that often emerges with energy healing is discussed within the context of transpersonal psychology.

7

THE PSYCHOENERGETIC PROCESS OF EMOTIONAL CLEARING AND TRANSFORMATION

In this chapter we consider the steps of the psychoenergetic healing sequence and the actual hand movements that the therapist uses to facilitate emotional clearing and transformation. We know that energy-oriented interventions can be a powerful tool for the healing of emotional wounds. They enhance the sensitivity and strengths that are already present in the counselor's repertoire, blending knowledge and skill into a healing art. As with many other adjunctive methods, clinical judgment is needed to discern their most appropriate use with selected clients.

INITIAL CONSIDERATIONS

We want to reiterate the importance of verbal and nonverbal rapport which creates the resonance for energy-related work. As we recall from Chapter 4, the energy fields of the client and therapist interact constantly. There is a flow of energy from the fuller, more focused field of the counselor to the depleted or imbalanced field of the client. If the therapist is not centered, the boundless flow from the Universal Energy Field will be restricted so that the client may receive only a small portion of what is actually available. In that case, the potential for change will be limited. On the other hand, if the receiver's field is more expanded than the therapist's, as sometimes happens when health care professionals are very tired, the client may dominate the interaction with the end result that there is little progress in reaching therapeutic goals.

Rapport can further be established by communicating about energy-related concepts at the level appropriate to the client. Since a growing number of health care consumers are familiar with energy healing concepts, they may ask specific questions about their fields or chakras. In such cases, it can be useful to provide simple explanations. It is best to avoid getting sidetracked into lengthy intellectual discussions. For clients who have no stated interest in energetic principles, the therapist can introduce the material briefly by suggesting that this work facilitates relaxation and includes hand movements above the client's physical body. (Informed consent is also advisable with any new or unusual modality, and is discussed more fully in Chapter 15.)

Another crucial aspect of rapport is in noting the client's affect and capacity for responding to visible hand movements in the energy field. With persons who are confused, actively decompensating, or very dissociated from their feelings, it may be best to omit hand motions because they might be misinterpreted. Our most valuable energetic resource is our ability to hold a centered focus with such clients. We recall the importance of setting our intent on behalf of the client and for the client's highest good. In addition, we can be creative by including internal imagery; for example, if a confused patient could benefit from gentle smoothing of the field, the therapist can image such a movement in the mind's eye. This may indirectly help the client to relax without arousing concern about hand gestures. We remember that psychoenergetic healing is basically nonlocal in nature; physical touch is not required. The therapist's intent, focus, and alignment with the boundless energy resources of the universe create the healing environment.

The therapist may choose to weave energetic interventions into her usual therapeutic maneuvers, or plan sessions in which only the healing sequence described here is followed (see the Summary at the end of the chapter). During energy healing sessions the client is fully clothed and seated comfortably in a chair or recliner. The therapist may be sitting or move quietly around the client while performing energetic assessment or intervention.

PERSONAL EMPOWERMENT

Understanding of energy field concepts gives us very practical ways of enhancing client self-awareness. For many people, it is a pleasant surprise to learn that they even have an energy field. Awareness of the human energy field establishes an experience of expanded consciousness and of being more than just a physical body with a limited identity. Something as simple as the energy field assessment can be a source of encouragement and support for the client. The idea of monitoring their own energy fields gives many clients a tremendous sense of personal choice and self-empowerment.

Joan was a client who suffered abuse in early childhood and was involved in a destructive relationship with her spouse when she came for counseling. Everything that had happened reinforced her sense of helplessness and powerlessness. Her counselor soon came to impasses in his attempts to convince Joan that she had any self-worth. Out of sheer desperation, he asked Joan to do the hand exercises described in Chapter 6 to sense her own energy field. Joan felt tingling between her hands almost immediately and responded with a look of delight. Next, she brought her hands over her body and noted temperature differences, feeling areas of warmth, especially over her heart. Her whole face lit up with the joy of experiencing herself in such a direct way. She literally had found a new way of relating to herself. From that day on, she knew she was "somebody." Centering on a regular basis and perceiving her energy field gave her a heightened sense of personal strength. Within several months she confronted her spouse, moved out, and began a healthier life on her own, trusting her own inner wisdom.

The assessment of the client's energy field provides useful information to the therapist about areas of blocked energy flow and the chakras most related to the constrictions in the field. If, for example, the first chakra is diminished, we can make educated guesses concerning related psychological issues. Aside from possible physical disorders related to stress, the healer can assume other emotions such as fear, survival, and safety issues linked to a lack of joy and vitality toward life. (Further possible psychological issues related to the root chakra are discussed in Chapter 5.)

Keeping the importance of rapport in mind, the helper may objectively share assessment information with the client if it is appropriate. Certainly, any comments must be free of judgment or criticism. Telling someone "Your first chakra is blocked" or "You must be afraid of something" would decidedly not be helpful ways to proceed. However, a statement such as "I find the area at the base of the spine low in energy. This sometimes relates to a sense of insecurity or fear. Does that have any meaning for you?" allows the client freedom to accept or deny the presence of these feelings. Regardless of the response, safety and trust issues have been raised. The client's awareness of these recurring themes will increase until he indicates readiness to address them.

It is essential that any feedback elicited from the energy field be presented in as neutral a fashion as possible. There should be no suggestion of content, projection of one's own material, or putting words in the client's mouth. We respect the client's inner process and self-esteem without any expectations or hidden agendas. Our intent is consistently set towards making energy available to the client for his self-healing.

SPONTANEOUS SURFACING OF UNRESOLVED MATERIAL

Often, clients will spontaneously access unrecognized or repressed material just as the therapist assesses the client's energy field. Assessment allows direct contact with a stored or embedded memory. For example, in the work with Betsy described in Chapter 2, the healer's sensing of the depleted area over the second chakra helped Betsy to connect with her core self-esteem issues. We also remember that the second chakra is associated with major emotional issues, such as choosing relationships, expressing sexuality, and being aware of feelings. It is logical that this was a blocked area in Betsy's field since she had major issues around her promiscuous sexual past and low self-esteem.

Dora Kunz speaks of the pervasive quality of the emotional energy field as connecting us to the ". . . dynamic patterns or configurations within which change is continually taking place" (Kunz, 1991, p. 26). She further describes her visual perceptions that include sensing the predominant color and symbols of trauma in the client energy field. Based on her intuitive assessments, Ms. Kunz could then indicate the most appropriate areas for psychological follow-up.

Another example from our extensive files comes to mind. Frank had just completed 18 months of behavioral cognitive therapy. Having read about energy healing, he wanted to have a few psychoenergetic sessions to round out his course of therapy. When the therapist passed her hands over his legs and feet, he winced in pain. Within moments, a turbulent memory flashed before his eyes: he was 2½ years old and being bullied by his older brother who was mowing the lawn. In a fit of rage, the brother ran over his legs and feet with the family lawnmower. This early childhood trauma had never been addressed emotionally, although extensive physical care was required after the accident. "I haven't thought of that in years and certainly not in my previous therapy. Why did it come up here so quickly?" he asked.

As he explored the incident and the circumstances surrounding it, Frank uncovered a whole barrage of resentments associated with the older brother's ongoing insults. Frank never felt worthy of his parents' love because they basically ignored the problematic sibling rivalry. Even though he received better grades in school, he always felt somehow diminished by his older brother. The relationship was strained and inadequate; the parents' blindness to the problem made him doubt his own perceptions and he perceived the situation as crazy-making. Until his experience with energy work, he never realized how much fear and anger he was holding toward his only sibling.

Frank was surprised how quickly all this related material surfaced once the most traumatizing memory had surfaced. Now that it was available, he began releasing many related issues, one by one, while the therapist helped to clear the affected areas of the energy field. To facilitate clearing of the emotional wound, the therapist encouraged Frank to come up with an image or action that would help him complete the healing. Frank knew that he and his brother needed to meet and talk about all that had occurred. Afterward, Frank did indeed contact his brother, who was deeply remorseful about the lawnmower incident. They were able to talk as adults and make amends with each other. Many other associated family incidents came to light that could also be discussed. In time, Frank and his brother became friends for the first time.

PATTERNS OF BLOCKAGE IN THE ENERGY FIELD

As suggested in our earlier discussion, all kinds of emotional material can become embedded in the energy field. This results in a constriction of the usual flow of energy that connects the centers of consciousness to the Universal Energy Field and to the energetic layers of the individual's aura.

Since all trauma to the physical body cuts through the layers of the field, we can expect a disturbance in the outer layers of the aura, notably the emotional, mental, and spiritual dimensions. The physical wound may close with a scar and fractures can recalcify, but the person involved in the trauma may feel his life is forever altered in some way. Even more benign forms of physical trauma such as diagnostic or surgical procedures, can result in a sense of emptiness and depression long after the surgeon's stitches have been removed. Each of us has worked with clients who say, "I've never felt the same since my operation." From an energetic perspective, we conclude that the layers of the energy field have not resealed themselves. Emotional reintegration is needed to release the effects of the trauma and to rebalance the energy field in these instances.

Emotional trauma can be even more devastating to the human energy field than physical injury. Because the wound is not overtly visible, many persons suffer from emotional injuries that have never been resolved. Childhood events, occurring when we are most vulnerable and when we do not have adequate coping resources, can and do cause hidden effects resulting in lifelong feelings of diminished self-worth. When the original event is not remembered or is suppressed, it is even more difficult to ascertain the cause.

Such was the case with Frank and his brother. The unwitting parents probably thought the injury was healed when the scar tissue formed over the physical wounds. However, as therapists, we know that such childhood incidents often become part of ongoing emotional pain, creating a distorted system of beliefs about the world. We call these faulty beliefs "complexes" that influence whole patterns of thinking, with widening levels of distrust, projection, and prejudice. The doubts and limiting beliefs generate filters that distort accurate perception of the world. In energy field language, we consider such emotional and mental distortions blocks to healthy energy flow. These constrictions can be present throughout a whole lifetime without ever being addressed, preventing clients from reaching their fullest potential.

Recent trauma, whether it is emotional or psychological in nature, causes similar impediments to the energy flow in the field. The main difference is that recent trauma is usually more accessible, remembered by the client, and available for resolution. Also, the client's resources are quite different as an adult and can be drawn on to assist in the clearing of the pattern.

EMOTIONAL CLEARING

In the language of traditional therapy, when an emotional block is remembered in its full emotional intensity, a *catharsis* (release of the emotional tension) takes place. Often, all that is needed to connect with the intense feelings stored in the subconscious is permission from the therapist. At other times, encouragement and statements of overt support from the facilitator further assist the client. As therapists, we must be sure we are comfortable with abreactive material and the expression of usually forbidden thoughts, such as murderous fantasies. Any discomfort on the therapist's part can be communicated to the healee through the interactive energy fields and inhibit the client's full expression of the emotion.

As the client lets the emotion flow out by crying, yelling, coughing, laughing, or moving expressively in the safe environment of the therapeutic setting, the emotional intensity of the traumatic event is matched. With the release of the energetically held feelings, the client can move to new insights for resolution. Frank followed emotional release with ideas about approaching his brother. The event that was literally "stuck" in the past was brought into the present. From there, new action and integration were possible.

Exploring Secondary Gains

The energetic approaches presented here blend well with traditional therapeutic maneuvers to facilitate emotional release and enrich them by offering deeper, nonverbal clearing of blocked patterns. As in all effective therapy, it is very helpful to ask the client to go back in personal history to explore earlier sources of the distressing emotion and the possible consequences of releasing the pattern. The client is encouraged to ask himself, "What would be the result if I fully give up this emotional pain?" If there indeed are perceptible consequences, it is important to explore the possible secondary gains associated with the held pattern and address them directly.

Accessing the Positive Intent

Another very useful intervention is to assist the client in connecting with the positive intent behind his choices, which may have included feeling like a victim, or being the martyr, avoider, or loner. We help the client to understand that many choices made in early life were based on limited information and often under perceived threat from a powerful adult. Resonating with the positive intent behind early decisions allows the client to attract and create new, more effective patterns to achieve his positive goal.

Externalizing the Event or Person

Another helpful tool in the therapeutic resource kit is the externalizing of an internal event. In classical Gestalt therapy (Perls, 1969) the incomplete form, or *gestalt*, of a past time can be brought into the present by bringing the central figure from the past to mind and addressing that person directly. For example, in the safety of the therapist's office, Frank practiced talking to his bullying brother as an empowered adult. With this practice, Frank opened the door to speaking directly without feeling lost, dominated, or insecure when he later approached his brother.

Another possible way to assist clients is by encouraging them to externalize the younger, and usually more distressed self of the past. This is especially useful when the client is judgmental about his prior behavior. Using this method, Betsy addressed her younger self, the troubled, pregnant teenager of the past, to come to a better understanding of herself. With the aid of her current adult awareness and the counselor's support, Betsy could explore the dynamics of the difficult history and bring in a quality of forgiveness. This technique is akin to the inner child work that has become very popular recently in dealing with dissociated, unloved, or addicted parts of oneself. As an additional resource, the client has opportunity to receive verbal input and encouragement from the therapist throughout the dialogue.

Alliance with Fair Witness

There is a witness awareness that emerges when clients face unsavory past events with nonjudgmental support. In the energetic alliance between healer and healee, grief, terror, and rage can pass through without engulfing or overwhelming the client. He starts to sense that he is more than his past, ". . . not being that stuff from the past," as one client recently said. Disidentification from compelling past trauma is an essential part of the healing process.

Often, connecting to one's Higher Self also emerges with this work, a sense of being greater than our temporary human dramas and opening to a wider perspective. When clients consciously face issues with support and allow for release work, they gain a sense of trust in their own wisdom and begin to look very differently at their lives.

Ways of Facilitating Emotional Clearing

The therapist can assist the client's connecting with the stored, blocked patterns by gently moving her hands back and forth above the area that is constricted or depleted. Traumatic events that relate to one or more of the energy centers show up as palpable irregularities in the field on assessment. More emphatic hand movement in these areas of the client's field may include unforming or loosening the embedded pattern and pulling out the clogged material, as if to sweep it away. Encouraging the client to give strong expulsive breaths, sounds, or movements as part of his release process is an additional resource.

Clearing of the entire energy field, or a specific part, is the essential energetic intervention that creates the psychic opening for the client to develop new perspectives and change. Synonyms for this kind of maneuver used by energy healers are unruffling (Krieger, 1993), unforming, dissolving, releasing, pulling out, expulsing, or discharging. The intent is to dissipate the blocked material and to facilitate emotional freeing and mental clarity.

EMOTIONAL FILLING AND TRANSFORMATION

After clearing, there is a temporary energetic void; the client's field is very receptive to new options and perceptions at this time. Transformation becomes a possibility. For example, as an intense emotional energy pattern is released, forgiveness can occur. This usually does not mean contacting the specific, external individual concerned but rather letting go of the energy form, the emotional entanglement of anger, resentment, hurt, or self-blame associated with the conflict, and seeing the whole event from a new perspective.

The client's perception of himself and others changes as forgiveness increases. To use one analogy, the half empty glass of water is now seen as half full. The person structures his thinking, his imagery, and his sense of place in the world differently. Dr. Leonard Laskow describes three progressive transformational steps by analogy (1992, p. 222): 1) switching from a noisy, overly commercial radio channel to a more enjoyable frequency, such as an FM station with soothing music; 2) making your own music, or writing and producing the movie of your life; and 3) moving beyond limited thinking to become co-creative, aligning with Universal Consciousness.

Modulating the client's energy flow to a new, more harmonious frequency is accomplished as the therapist holds her hands still over the area that has been cleared. This allows for a filling of the emptied area with whatever insight is needed to bring balance and harmony to the client's field. It is as if the inflow of the client's new awareness is stabilized and validated through the therapist's respectful silence. During this time, the therapist holds her focused intent for the highest good. The client may report internal imagery or specific insights as part of the integration. Often, a decrease of somatic symptoms and discomfort is noted. The healer can also encourage the client to take long slow breaths allowing for inflow of new energy, literally "to be inspired."

There are many synonyms used by intuitive healers for this modulation of energy. Some speak of transferring energy, while others use words such as filling, reforming, transforming, expanding, aligning, repatterning, or balancing the field.

The two basic energetic maneuvers—*clearing* of bound, constricted material and *modulation* to a more harmonious frequency—may be repeated as often as needed. At times, one issue is released to open the path for other related issues to emerge. A smoothing of the entire field, which is shaped like an enveloping rainbow arch or large egg, completes the energetic sequence. At the end of the session, as the client discusses his inner changes, he naturally becomes more grounded and connected to ordinary, consensus reality. It is wise to allow ample time for complete reorientation before the client leaves the healing session.

THE PSYCHOENERGETIC HEALING PROCESS

We can now formulate a sequence of energy-related maneuvers that can be used by therapists to facilitate emotional healing. Briefly, the steps are as follows:

1. Assess the client's entire energy field and note areas of disturbance or depletion, especially over each energy center.
2. While moving the hands over a depleted or imbalanced part of the field, ask the client what image, color or memory comes to mind.
3. As specific material is brought forth, support the client by encouraging full expression of related emotions.
4. After the initial emotional release, help the client to disidentify from the historical material by externalizing the associated person or event.
5. Assist emotional clearing by moving the hands away from the congested area with broad sweeping, releasing hand motions. Let the client support the release with strong, expulsive breaths or sounds.
6. Encourage the client to reconnect with his resources for resolving the material in the present in a creative, congruent manner while at the same time, modulating energy over the related energy centers.
7. Complete the sequence by balancing and smoothing the entire energy field, allowing the client to integrate the work by viewing it from the perspective of his higher Self. Let the client experience a deep inflow of energy and inspiration with full relaxation breaths.
8. Allow the client to share his internal experience, making sure he is oriented to consensus reality before leaving your presence.

DISCUSSION

To review the sequence in more detail, first we consider the assessment of the client's energy field. What is the overall condition of the field? Does it feel symmetrical and smooth? Does it have a "bouncy" or vibrant feeling? Is it asymmetrical, rough, uneven in temperature, or "flat" in certain areas? The condition of each chakra can also be sensed, allowing us to know where there are specific constrictions linked to psychological concerns.

Some clients are very interested in learning the results of the assessment and are able to give additional related information about themselves. Others will be less active and simply let the therapist assist them with relaxation.

After energy field assessment and a brief psychosocial interview, we can formulate a psychoenergetic diagnosis (a suggested outline for psychoenergetic assessment can be found in Appendix B). This may be stated in brief, energetic terms, as ". . . energy field disturbance in relation to specific energy center #___" or include a description of the overall quality of the field noting areas of asymmetry. The energy field disturbance (NANDA, 1995–1996) may also relate to repeated physical injuries throughout the client's lifetime. Thus, we may note an "energy center of causation," an area to which many problems are related.

Together, the healer and healee identify areas for internal work after the therapist has noted energetic assessment and lifelong patterns related to the energy centers. The therapist next asks the client to be as comfortable as possible in the chair or recliner and encourages a more relaxed state of consciousness. There are, of course, numerous ways to encourage the client to be calmer and more focused. One means is to suggest that the client release tension and worries with the out-breath and allow new resources from the Universal Energy Field to enter with the in-breath. The therapist then allows the hands to move slowly over each chakra, beginning at the root, focusing especially over any chakra that was distorted or depleted during assessment.

At this time, the client may spontaneously share an image, a color, or sound that comes to her. Otherwise, the facilitator can simply ask, "What image, perception, or memory comes to you now?" Often, this is enough for the client to connect with a significant unresolved issue. Another option is to have the client verbalize a statement out loud that is relevant to the depleted energy center. An affirmation such as "I feel my vitality," or "I enjoy being alive in this body" will feel incongruent if the root chakra is indeed blocked. A half-hearted, doubtful verbalization in a low voice tone would be a clue to the therapist that this is not the client's truth at that moment. The incongruence between the statement and the client's current affect offers ample material for further exploration. For instance, the therapist could ask, "Who or what keeps you from being fully alive and vital at this time?"

There are additional ways of encouraging clients to become more aware of half-truths or subtle dissociated parts. One is to have the healee repeat the affirmation that does not quite fit until inner tension builds. This augmented tension facilitates emotional release. Another is to follow the slightest movement in the body, such as a tense jaw, a clenched fist, or an involuntary foot movement. Encouraging the client to exaggerate this movement can put him in touch with the underlying emotional tension.

As soon as the discontinuity is brought to mind, the helper can assist the client by externalizing either the person or circumstance that seems to prohibit full vitality and aliveness. Externalizing the person, the past experience, or dissociated inner part allows the client to express feelings and to release the blocked emotion. Throughout the session, the therapist supports the client by gently moving hands over the blocked area of the energy field to assist the clearing process.

In contrast to the many therapies which see emotional release as an endpoint, the psychoenergetic approach continues. After emotional clearing, the next step is to connect with new options and larger energy fields by tapping into the higher Self, the love and wisdom of the transpersonal dimension. By holding the hands over the cleared area, the therapist facilitates the client's connection to his greater resources while modulating, or transferring, energy. In addition, she can utilize the affirmations or positive statements related to optimum functioning of a specific chakra. For example, when tension and anger from the root chakra are released, the client can begin to affirm the new thinking pattern: "I deserve to feel alive;" "I sense and enjoy my body;" or "The Universe supports my physical being."

Many times the client will know exactly what is needed to move forward once the block is removed. It was clear to Frank, in our example, that he needed to contact his brother, to discuss their past, and to heal the broken relationship. With this came a sense of personal power and a gratifying feeling of wholeness.

Clients will often connect with images about new options or a sense of inner peace that expands to self-transcendence. Because imagery and the transpersonal domain are such important components of the healing process, we explore these resources for enhancement of the client's well-being in the next two chapters.

SUMMARY

The most important aspect of adding energetic approaches to psychotherapy is that when the therapist is in a truly centered state, she helps to ensure that nothing is imposed on the client. There is no projection or leading of the client. Unlike many modalities in which the therapist may feel compelled to direct or influence the proceedings, the client selects themes from his own psychological makeup as memories or images surface.

In emotional clearing, the client actually experiences sensations, movement, and release through his body and energy field, appreciating what it means to be free from constrictions that were locked in the body/mind. The unburdening may include cognitive awareness or it may simply feel similar to the relief after a heavy weight is lifted. The expression of pent-up emotion usually comes readily with the therapist's supportive presence.

The energetic repatterning, or filling, through modulation allows the client to experience imagery and an expanded perspective in relation to the conflicted material. From this higher level of functioning, integration and insight can flow more easily.

REFERENCES

Krieger, D. *The Therapeutic Touch*. Englewood Cliffs, NJ: Prentice-Hall Publishing Co., 1979.

Kunz, D. *The Personal Aura*. Wheaton, IL: Quest Books, 1991.

Laskow, L. *Healing with Love*. San Francisco, CA: HarperCollins, 1992.

North American Nursing Diagnosis Association. "NANDA Nursing Diagnoses: Definitions and Classification 1995-1996." Philadelphia, PA.

Perls, F. *Gestalt Therapy Verbatim*. Lafayette, CA: Real People Press, 1969.

8 PSYCHOENERGETIC IMAGERY

Imagery is a readily available tool that can be applied anytime, anywhere. In this chapter, we examine the role of imagery in relation to multilevel healing. When speaking of imagery, we refer not only to visual, but also to olfactory, taste, tactile, and auditory representations, as well as the full use of our imaginations to enhance healing potential (Achterberg et al., 1994; Shames, 1996). The following example shows how imagery can be used in conjunction with energy healing.

William's Story: The Glands Party

William was a 67-year-old writer recently diagnosed with inoperable colon cancer. He viewed his diagnosis as a "hit below the belt." Much of his life had revolved around his creative endeavors. Having never married, he prided himself on his talents as an illustrator and with his sexual artistry. He had a history of intimate relations with countless beautiful women in his small, open-minded community.

When she first started to work with William, the therapist noted his depleted, constricted heart center on assessment. His response was that he was mending a "broken heart" because he had recently ended a long-term relationship. He was angry at himself for having chosen such an inappropriate person to love. As he discussed his goals for therapy, he stated that he would like to incorporate imagery into his healing program.

For the first two sessions, William and his therapist explored avenues of addressing his illness and broken heart. The therapist also introduced energy healing concepts. By the third session, he envisioned bright, rich colors which corresponded to the chakras being treated when she gently modulated energy in his field. It became evident that his inner life was very colorful, as one might anticipate in an artist. Several sessions later, he was bathing each part of the body in the colors of the corresponding chakra, while the therapist voice-guided him through the process of the chakra meditation described in Chapter 5.

At one point, the therapist suggested William expand his imagery to include the specific endocrine glands associated with each energy center. When her hands were placed over his lower limbs, she suggested that he see the entire area glowing in rich, colorful red. She then recommended that he picture the adrenal glands (endocrine glands) associated with the first chakra. She asked him what he saw, and he described an image of bright red adrenals, holding cocktail glasses filled with carrot and beet juice, toasting and having a merry time. They then moved on to the second chakra, with her hands lightly moving over the hip area, while he imaged bathing his gonads in a brilliant orange. He found it especially helpful to inundate the pelvis with the bright orange light because this was the identified area related to his physical and emotional problems. He also pictured the colon filling with orange sunlight, revitalizing itself, looking full and restored. Chakra by chakra, they worked together in similar fashion.

When all the endocrine glands were bathed in their specific healing color, William spontaneously decided to have them all meet together for a colorful party, where each was laughing, jovial, and healthy. His belly jiggled with laughter as he used his artist's imagination to uplift his spirits and invigorate his energy field. Afterwards, he remarked that he had not laughed so hard in many months. Most noticeable was the return of color to his face, enhanced by a sense of serenity.

The mixture of psychotherapy with imagery and energy healing proved to be a potent combination, opening the floodgates to repressed emotions. Within a short time, deep issues surfaced. He shared worry about not having sexual relations since his diagnosis, although he had several opportunities. When asked why he had not chosen to act, he became very sad and spoke softly.

"I'm almost 70, I'm broke, and I have colon cancer. Who would want to be with me?" His grief was apparent. Loss of sexuality can be devastating to anyone, but for him, it was monumental. He had built a powerful image of himself based on his ability to communicate through sexual expression, and now this avenue seemed closed for the first time.

Despite the fact that he was handsome, intelligent, and humorous, he was disheartened because of the cancer diagnosis which felt like a cruel twist of fate. His poetry, which appeared in local newspapers, became progressively dark and sarcastic.

His energy healing sessions allowed him a reprieve from the intense reality of his inner turmoil. He enjoyed lying on the recliner in the therapy room and relaxing. His life felt stressful and hectic, and this quiet time provided him with a place to be nurtured. He often became very peaceful when he created a new scenario each week, combining imagery with energy healing. Many times, he laughed through much of the session, which in itself is powerful medicine.

In their work together, the therapist often chose to use interactive imagery techniques, rather than guided visualization, which is more directive. After the initial shock of a difficult diagnosis, most people seem to feel empowered by having several options from which to choose. For them, selecting their own images for healing is helpful. Other clients feel overwhelmed, and require strong direction from the counselor. It is valuable to pay attention to the approach that is best for each client, keeping in mind that the need for independent choice-making or specific guidance may vary from week to week. The therapist must remain flexible, following the client's needs at a given time to direct the session.

IMAGERY TERMINOLOGY

A major impact of counseling is derived from our ability to work with mental images. Often, clients are either projecting their concerns into the future or reflecting back on memories from the past through their own imagery. Clients will share vivid dreams or fears which convey material from the various layers of consciousness. The therapy setting, usually a quiet office that is devoid of any specific references to the client's life, allows work on personal issues through the active imagination.

When we add energy balancing to psychotherapy, clients will often report physical sensations in direct response to the work. It is useful to address these sensations, using all the senses to enrich the client's experience and provide him with opportunity for integration.

There are many terms related to the use of imagery. Some are used interchangeably, and although there is no consensus among the varying definitions, each can assist in our understanding. Exploring imagery expands our resources for multidimensional healing, supporting our efforts to restore and revitalize the client's energy field.

What Is an Image?

Images come to us from all the senses. Although we think of images as being associated with sight, we actually perceive them through a variety of senses, depending upon which ones are most readily accessible and familiar. An image is actually a thought with sensations attached, a mental representation of something which may or may not exist in the present moment. We sometimes have a feeling, smell, sound, or taste prior to forming a visual image. Some individuals are predominantly kinesthetic and feel physical sensations easily. Each person has a unique blend of sensory responsiveness to environmental stimuli. As life experiences accumulate, a single image, such as the smell of sage, can evoke recall of multiple associations.

Images, therefore, are symbolic representations that describe inner experience. For example, we have learned much about ancient civilizations through their symbolic depictions on cave walls. In modern times as well, symbols can activate intuitive thinking, permitting quick, insightful, and imaginative associations. These spontaneous images are less structured than analytical thinking because they incorporate the creative faculties of the mind. We have found that intuition becomes very active when we combine images with energy healing.

What Is Imagery?

The term *imagery* refers to a broad concept that involves thoughts and feelings simultaneously. In imagery, the image or symbol is combined with sensations and emotion. In William's example, the therapist supported his visualization of the colors associated with the chakras, which then led to the client's spontaneous imagery of the gland party, further triggering an emotional release that left them both laughing.

Therapeutic imagery applies to those instances when the client's natural imagination is utilized to direct the mind toward beneficial results and therapeutic goals.

Guided imagery is used to describe the experience of leading the subject to a positive response through the use of words, ideas, and symbols. Often, the scenario is richly painted and enhanced by the words of the therapist or helper.

Visualization was popularized by a number of self-help books, most notably Shakti Gawain's *Creative Visualization* (1983). Although the concept was intended to refer to all healing endeavors using imagery, visualization is most often associated with visual strategies. For this reason, the word *imagery* is more accurate to describe the broader concept that allows for helpful input from all the senses.

Interactive imagery is a further expansion of the concept, popularized in the last decade among health professionals through the teachings of the Academy for Guided Imagery co-directed by Martin Rossman, M.D. and David Bresler, Ph.D. (Rossman, 1987). This practice uses guided imagery, but allows the client to participate in the process, creating his or her own healing insights. It has proven to be a highly effective tool in which the client can become aware of internal guidance to activate states of well-being. The therapist helps to set the scene and holds an emotional safety net, while the client's subconscious mind invents the specific tools for healing. At the same time, the person's relaxation response is also activated.

JUNG'S CONCEPT OF SYMBOLISM

In 1964, Carl Jung published a landmark book, *Man and His Symbols*, which helped to shape new directions in psychotherapy. Prior to this publication, the bulk of information about our inner symbolic life, and its associations with the unconscious realm, remained with analysts and scholars. Jung's book awakened a wide readership to awareness of their own internal life, helping them to delve more deeply into their own psyches for personal answers.

Jung shed light on the importance of the intuitive, nonrational aspect of ourselves, and enticed us to explore the mystical side. Since the time of Rene Descarte at the end of the

seventeenth century, numerous efforts had been made to lo-
cate the human soul. Given that science could not physically
find the soul (despite the efforts of such brilliant anatomical
scientists as William Harvey) the soul came to be considered
less important than the body. As a result, people increasingly
viewed themselves as fragmented and compartmentalized.
This philosophy assigned a lesser status to the active imagination and greater status to rational thinking.

Jung, however, began to unravel the myth of the fragmented person, insisting that within all of us are stored memories, perhaps even from ancient times, that could be accessed
through exploring dreams, instincts, and daytime reverie. He
further distinguished between *sensation* which tells us that
something exists, *feeling* which informs us whether it is pleasant or not, *thinking* which identifies what it is, and *intuition*
which informs us of its source, its personal importance, and
possible future implications (Jung, 1964, p. 61).

In proceeding to explore the role of the psyche via symbols and myths, Jung eventually arrived at ways of working
with images. He believed that cultural images and natural symbols were used as communication tools in primitive societies.
Symbols and stories have been used throughout the ages to express eternal truth and innate wisdom. Jung called this shared
human consciousness by means of symbols the "collective unconscious." We might also think of this shared human memory
as a collective energy field that is accessible to everyone of us.

Jung further articulated the idea that, just as the body
stores its history, so the mind gathers and saves all images in
its vast reservoirs. This happens not only through conscious
language, but also through symbols, including unconscious archaic images stored in the psyche. He called these recurring
patterns *archetypes*. The archetype forms representations of a
theme, images that may vary in shape but are similar in basic
pattern. He further explained: "Only after I had familiarized
myself with alchemy did I realize that the unconscious is a
process, and that the psyche is transformed or developed by
the relationship of the ego to the contents of the unconscious.
In individual cases, that transformation can be read from
dreams and fantasies. In collective life it has left its deposit
principally in various religious systems and their changing
symbols" (Jung, 1964, p. 209).

The archetypes, therefore, are archaic remnants or primor-
dial images, originating in the subconscious mind. Instincts are

physiological urges perceived by the senses, whereas the archetypes can manifest themselves in fantasies and dreams and reveal their presence only through the use of symbolic images. For example, the universal symbol of a wise, nurturing caregiver is manifest in some form in every culture, primitive or sophisticated, around the world. This healer archetype is without specific origin but reflects a collective human experience.

According to Jung, "We can perceive the specific energy of archetypes when we experience the peculiar fascination that accompanies them. They seem to hold a special spell . . . but while personal complexes never produce more than a personal bias, archetypes create myths, religions, and philosophies that influence and characterize whole nations and epochs of history" (Jung, 1964, p. 79).

Thus, we come to understand how someone could be released from his sense of impotence and receive almost magical powers through identification with mythical heroes and their struggles. As client or therapist, this is the power we tap into when we assist clients in embarking on their healing journey. In essence, we create a safe place for delving into subconscious imagery and sparking creativity through dreams, images, and archetypes.

IMAGERY FOR PSYCHOENERGETIC COUNSELING

Counseling that blends imagery with energetic techniques is greatly enhanced and more effective. The client's participation in the interactive process is facilitated by moving from simple to more complex symbols. Thus, we begin with encouraging the client to relax through breathing exercises, move on to creating a safe and protected place, access images that fill in the client's missing experiences, and finally, incorporate inner guidance.

Relaxation to Connect with the Internal Energy Flow

The relaxation response was described extensively by Herbert Benson (1975) and refers to a psychophysiological state in which the parasympathetic nervous system is activated: muscles are relaxed, tension is released; blood pressure, heart rate, pulse and respirations are lowered; the brain shifts to the alpha brain wave pattern (signifying a deepened state of relaxation); and the parasympathetic nervous system is activated. This effects a balance with the sympathetic nervous system, the arousal mechanism, and allows for the body to engage in restorative patterns, rather than letting the "fight or flight" stress response predominate.

There are many ways to activate the relaxation response which facilitate the client's inner awareness of himself. One method is to start with relaxation of one body area, such as the feet, and then to gradually bring the sensation of warmth and relaxation to other parts of the body as well. This process is sometimes called *progressive relaxation.* Other ways to induce a more internally-focused state include alternately tensing and relaxing the muscle groups and breathing deeply. Imagery enhances the relaxation; for example, visualizing a bright blue sky at the beach, hearing gentle surf, smelling the ocean, and feeling the warm sun creates a much deeper sense of calm than simply relaxing various muscle groups.

"Breathing is a powerful physiological process. Many ancient traditions, including yoga, work with the breath to encourage energy flow. Energy can become blocked in numerous places in the body. Breathing can increase the energy flow and help to remove blockages" (Shames, 1996, p. 84). When we work with the breath, we are working with our life force, our energy. Therefore, focusing on the breath induces a relaxed state in the client as well as providing a direct experience of the unceasing flow of energy in the body.

Introducing work with the breath informs the client that he has the ability to use his own mechanisms—the breath and the mind—to nourish and support his soul. The following exercises, described in a way that the therapist could use to voice-guide the client, are two suggestions for increasing awareness of energy flow.

Exercise: Breathing to Feel the Flow of Internal Energy

1. Sit comfortably with feet flat on the ground, good support for the back, and belt loosened to allow for deep breathing.

2. Notice any part of the body that is uncomfortable and release the tension by moving or shaking out the discomfort.

3. Exhale fully, as if you were slowly blowing out a candle. Then exhale even more. Do this several times to clear out any tension, letting it flow out your hands and feet as well.

4. Bring your awareness to the in-breath, reminding yourself that this is an opportunity for renewal. As you exhale, further cleanse the whole body. As you inhale, bring in the new. Sense the ongoing cycle of releasing the old and bringing in the new.

5. Sense the revitalizing of your body through the cycle of the breath. Throughout the day, connect to the next breath whenever you feel tension; remind yourself of your inner resources for renewal with your breath.

Exercise: Breathing Through the Energy Centers

1. Sit or lie down in a comfortable position; clear out any tension with the breath.

2. Image connect to the earth with the soles of your feet. Sense the support of the earth's energy field, the predictable force of gravity, the beauty of nature around you, and the beauty of sunlight dancing on waves somewhere, even on a cloudy day.

3. Breathe in slowly and deeply through the nose, drawing in earth's energy and wisdom. As you exhale through the mouth, remind yourself that this is an opportunity to release any impediments, pain, sadness, or fear. Draw in strength and courage, and let go of anything that is stale or no longer helpful.

4. Sense the power of this inhaling and exhaling at the base of the spine, increasing your sense of aliveness.

5. Sense the clearing out of the old and the bringing in of the new in the lower abdomen, selecting whatever works for you and letting go of what does not.

6. Sense the in-breath and out-breath in the solar plexus area, feeling your power and ability to communicate effectively.

7. Breathe in a similar fashion through the upper energy centers of the heart, throat, brow, and crown. Sense the expansion of unconditional positive regard toward

self and others, your creativity, your compassion, and your alignment with your Higher Power.

8. Sense your entire energy field expanding with the breath, empowered through your own images of the centers. Gently return to full awareness feeling relaxed and refreshed.

Accessing Pleasant and Protective Experiences

Another easily learned tool for relaxation and enhancing positive feelings is to tap into the ability for storing pleasant memories and remembering a sense of comfort. Often, clients tend to focus on distressing situations and unpleasant emotions. The mind then sorts for earlier memories with similar sensations and negative emotional content. One method for countering such negativity quickly is to counterbalance with a pleasant memory or the sense of being safe and protected. This is not intended to distract the client from needed emotional work, but to help client awareness of alternatives which make it easier to cope with negativity and to increase restorative potential in the energy field.

Exercise: Creating a Safe Place

1. When you feel tired or frazzled, imagine going to a place that is special and safe so you can gather your energy again and feel stronger.

2. Begin by sitting comfortably and releasing tension as you exhale slowly several times.

3. Now, think of a place in nature that you remember as being special to you, or one you have seen in a picture or dream.

4. *See* the colors of the special place: notice the time of day, and notice the sunlight or clouds. *Hear* the sounds associated with this place: the birds and the wind moving through the trees. *Smell* the freshness of the breeze, the flowers, or woods. *Feel* the relaxation and comfort of this special place: feel the warmth of the sun and the gentle breeze.

5. Allow a pleasant thought to emerge, such as "I am at peace; I am loved and supported."

6. Let yourself return to full awareness feeling refreshed and aware of new options.

Exercise: The Protective Bubble

1. After relaxing yourself with the breath, envision yourself within a protective bubble.

2. Allow your imagination to expand the image as you consider some suggestions. The protective bubble might feel similar to a warm cocoon, surrounded by calming music. Or it might appear as a pink or white sheath of protective light.

3. Affirm the existence of this protective barrier, and envision it, seeing it in whatever way you wish. You might see a painter on a ladder, painting an egg-shaped bubble around you in full glorious color. You may picture an animal guide working with you to maintain the protective bubble. The supportive structure could even be formed by a child blowing a huge balloon from a wand which encircles and encapsulates your entire being.

4. You might wish to make your bubble semipermeable, so that the small, light molecules of love and positive emotion can move back and forth, whereas darker, or threatening energy is held back. The protective bubble allows negative thoughts and emotions to be reflected back to their source so they are not absorbed.

5. Imagine walking protected in this bubble whenever you need it in your work or other settings. Appreciate your creativity in working with this bubble before returning to full awareness.

There are multiple ways for counselors and therapists to stimulate the creative imagination of clients. It is possible to introduce these techniques by first inviting the client to participate in a relaxation exercise, such as the ones presented above. It is also valuable to present the experience within the client's frame of reference. In fact, much of the art of therapeutic interaction is in its presentation. The words "imagery" or "energy healing" may activate an unconscious response because of prior programming, whereas the word "relaxation" evokes a comforting image for almost everyone. In clients' stressful lives, relaxation is recognized as a powerful antidote to accidents and exhaustion.

We can support the client's feeling of safety by teaching about the layers of the energy field (discussed in Chapter 4). Understanding that the body is the most dense part of the human energy field, clients can begin to appreciate their own multidimensional qualities. They can envision the etheric layer, the emotional layer, the mental layer, and the spiritual layer as further outreaches of their own indomitable spirit. Each layer can be strengthened and intensified to enhance the feeling of protection and support. The layers can further be reinforced with mental imagery or physical hand movements to smooth areas that are uneven or depleted. In this manner, the person can feel safer and more protected, genuinely loved and nurtured.

Externalizing the Problem

Another useful approach when confronting a challenge or problem is to have the client imagine a conflict to be well outside her energy field. This is a form of useful dissociation that allows the client to disconnect from being overly enmeshed with an anxiety-producing situation for a time, sufficiently long to consider alternative solutions.

For example, if the client is conflicted about a relationship, we can encourage her to see the challenging person sitting in front of her. The client may reinforce the layers of her field as a protective envelope to feel safer and in control. A further expansion of this concept is to have the client dialogue with the person, imagining a variety of responses. The client may need to rage or otherwise express her feelings, and to clearly set boundaries by letting the person know what is unacceptable. She might state her needs, while feeling safe in this more objective position.

Often, clients report that externalizing the problem in this way has eased the situation without actually needing to confront the individual in question. Simply changing one's own inner process becomes an act of empowerment.

Another option for externalizing the problem situation is to have the client take on the perspective of being the counselor. It is sometimes easier to imagine what a wise counselor would say, and then apply those ideas as a personal option. At times, the client might need to take the problem and dispose of it, perhaps locking it in a trunk or sinking it into the trash. This is especially effective if the problem is something which cannot be changed. This kind of imagery enables one to stop obsessing or feeling helpless and to move forward.

Creating Nurturing Parents

The growing literature on addictions and codependency has popularized the concept of the "inner child." Since many clients can relate to this framework, release from the tyranny of harmful parenting can be enhanced by adding inner child imagery to energetic interventions.

For example, if a client is feeling sad or angry about parental abuse, we can suggest that she release the birth parents to another realm, a place where they might find the help they need to heal their own wounding. The client can use the process we have described to externalize them, maybe even place them on a balloon or space ship, and direct their release in whatever manner feels productive.

The next step would be to have the client make contact with her inner child of the past, comforting and nurturing herself to facilitate inner healing. The therapist assists by moving gently in the client's field, perhaps in areas of congestion, or sitting by the client, holding protective energy, while the client searches for more nurturing parents. The therapist can voice-guide or suggest that the client envision parents walking toward her who then behave in the way that is needed to assist healing of the old wound. To round out the imagery, the client can articulate what is happening, what each person is doing, how it makes her feel, and perhaps even express gratitude for the nurturing parents. We can encourage the client to feel the effects of the caring parents' love in the physical body, and throughout all the layers of her field. At the same time the client can breathe deeply, releasing any places of stored hurt, and replenishing herself with the vital life force of nourishing energy.

Ultimately, we not only teach our clients these skills, but we empower them with tools for reparenting themselves. Clients can further be encouraged to view movies in their mind, seeing themselves as a successful protagonist or as a wise healer. They can envision themselves mastering their lives and challenges supported by a team of therapists, healers, or angels. All of these techniques can be expanded in numerous ways with the client's own unique imagery, and by facilitating energy flow with the breath.

Imagining the Picture of Health

One of the greatest benefits of using imagery with energy-related tools is that we can work with people suffering from illness and medical conditions without having to use medication or invasive procedures. For example, it is possible to access inner wisdom, perhaps finding the answers to painful health challenges, by helping the client to create her personal picture of health and then to move into her picture.

In making a picture of health and wholeness, clients can activate their own self-healing skills. In today's changing health care practice, clients increasingly recognize that if they are to become well, they must be advocates on their own behalf. We can inspire them by providing the support needed to develop their confidence and tenacity.

Exercise: The Picture of Health

1. Sit or lie down comfortably, releasing any tension as you exhale.

2. Imagine a large chart or map in front of you that represents your body. Scan the body map from head to toe, noticing any areas where your energy is congested or blocked. These areas might appear fuzzy or gray in color while the healthy, flowing areas are pink and clear.

3. Feeling the inflow of the healing breath and life force, move your attention to the areas that were congested and gradually let them become enlivened with your breath and focused intent.

4. Allow yourself to see the whole body in balance and harmony in a glow of the color you most like at this time.

5. Return to full awareness, continuing to feel the flow of more balance in your whole being.

Meeting the Inner Guide

The journey of the soul is an on-going one. One of the most meaningful tools for assisting the inner journey is to introduce the client to ways of finding his own inner healer. Twelve-step programs have been successful for a great number of people, helping them to feel less alone in their struggles against addictive thought patterns and behavior. Early on in these programs, participants are encouraged to connect to their Higher Power, or whatever concept assists them to expand to the nonlocal Mind. This concept elevates their thinking beyond the ego self to a more expanded vista, one in which the sufferer is no longer alone. The form of such vision is quite personal, ranging from the concept of a supreme being to images from the power of nature. While the higher resources imagined can adopt an infinite number of forms, their purpose is universal. People, when connected to their higher resources, are reminded—often through an externalized image—of their own innate wisdom and gifts. Our work as helpers is to reconnect clients with the power that is already within them awaiting their recall.

For most of us, a daily commitment is required to find higher guidance and live from it. This process allows the client to continually develop her internal relationship with self. The qualities of the inner guide include patience, unconditional love, nonjudgmental attitude, honesty, wisdom, compassion, and optimism.

The act of meeting one's inner guide can happen quickly for some, and very slowly for others. It can also be unexpectedly emotional at times. When a therapist of our acquaintance went to a beginning lecture on this topic years ago, she was sitting in the front row of a large auditorium. The speaker had set aside the last ten minutes of his presentation to give the group a brief experience of meeting inner guidance. As he voice-guided through a quick introduction, the healer had a strong image of her favorite grandmother who had died years ago standing in front of her, smiling and speaking to her. The image was so real that it took her by surprise and she burst out crying. Though the entire experience was extremely brief, it was deeply felt and significant.

Exercise: Finding the Inner Guide

1. Prepare by going mentally to your safe place. Eliminate possible distractions such as unplugging the phone and hanging a "Do Not Disturb" sign on the door of your room.

2. As you breathe and relax, let go of tension and envision your muscles relaxing. Pay attention to the

beauty and peace of your surroundings by carefully listening for sounds, feelings, temperature differences, smells, and other sensations. From this alert mental state, imagine that a being is coming toward you to bring you a message.

3. Allow the image to form as you see someone on the horizon walking toward you. It may or may not be human; some people relate more easily to an animal or a being from the angelic realm. Rather than trying to imagine who it is, simply allow the person or animal to arrive, seeing the feet first and then scanning upward.

4. As you sit quietly, notice the arrival of the messenger in great detail. Allow yourself to ask one or more questions related to current challenges in your daily life.

5. Pay close attention to the messages, words, gestures, or advice; ask more questions as you exhale sending out the breath, and allow the answers to come with the next inspiration.

6. Give thanks for the contact with the messenger. Agree to meet again at a given time, then watch as the creature or person leaves.

7. With several deep breaths, once again become aware of your feet on the floor, the room in which you are sitting, and any sounds or sensations in the environment. Keep a journal of these messages from inner guidance to help and strengthen your sense of internal dialogue.

William's Story Continued: The Inner Guide

We now return to the continuation of William's story, the client whose glands party enlivened his energy therapy sessions. The therapist's goal in working with William was to help him access his inner wisdom as quickly as possible because of his progressive cancer and limited lifetime. Whenever he came to the office, he would jump into the recliner and breathe deeply. As the therapist cleared his energy field, his sense of relaxation was palpable. When he had reached a very peaceful frame of mind, she invited him to take an inner journey. She spoke softly, encouraging him to imagine himself in a place that felt safe and protected.

She then asked him to envision someone coming toward him, a figure off in the distance. He knew it could be a person, an animal, or even a mythological creature. When he saw who was approaching, the therapist asked him to have the being sit down across from him and gaze gently into his eyes. William had the opportunity to dialogue with it and to ask any questions that might help him to heal. He spent quiet time listening closely.

After several minutes, William sat up and chuckled. He then explained what had transpired. When he was asked to envision an image, he saw a little boy coming toward him. Realizing that it was only a child, he tried to conjure up an image of something more powerful. He wanted to see a bear, his animal totem, and with great effort, he superimposed the image of a bear on top of the child. He was surprised, however, to notice that the little boy did not go away. The child merely slipped into the background, waiting patiently. When William invited the bear to sit with him, they looked into each others' eyes, but the bear would not talk with him. When William asked his questions, the bear just sat there, staring. Finally, the little boy in the background could not stand it any longer, and came stomping out from behind the tree. "Don't you understand!" the child exclaimed, "I was sent to you. I am the one with the answers you seek!"

When William finally realized that the child carried the wisdom he sought, he asked the many questions in his heart, and received inventive, powerful advice. He learned how he could revise his schedule to be less hurried and ways of utilizing nutrients to maintain well-being as much as possible. The child suggested his writing could become lighter, more playful; each day could be a gift for his full enjoyment. In sharing these insights with the therapist, William was animated, laughing, and obviously surprised at the creativity of his internal life. He realized how symbolic the entire session was: he was often trying to superimpose his will to make things appear as he thought they should be, rather than accepting his first intuitive hunch.

He left the session feeling light and bouncy, with a sense of wonder and joviality that he had not experienced for many months. He was reminded of life's magic and mystery which invited him to approach the last days of his life looking through the eyes of a child. He also felt more connected to his own playful child, an aspect of himself that had been neglected since he received his ominous diagnosis. William felt restored and replenished, ready to face the demands of his life with a renewed sense of courage and dignity.

SUMMARY

We have explored the valuable role of mental imagery in healing. Through the use of positive imaging, we can help affect the client's energy field, affirm life-enhancing imagery through creative use of the breath, connect to pleasant memories and a safe place, sense the protective layers of the energy field, and envision a protective bubble. We can further assist our clients in finding internal resources to supply the missing dimension of looking at a problem objectively, experiencing nurturing parents, and meeting the inner guide.

In addition, we are responsible for maintaining the integrity of our own field as therapists. We can expand our fields, through images and centered intent, so that we can effectively reach the client and support his process. Beyond planning and implementing therapeutic interventions, we are models of power and vitality while we support clients in activating their internal resources.

REFERENCES

Achterberg, J., Dossey, B., and Kolkmeier, L. *Rituals of Healing: Using Imagery for Health and Wellness.* New York: Bantam Books, 1994.

Gawain, S. *Creative Visualization.* Berkeley, CA: DeVorss Publishing Co., 1983.

Jung, C. *Man and His Symbols.* London: Aldus Books, 1964.

Jung, C. *Memories, Dreams, Reflections.* New York: Vintage Books, 1961.

Rossman, M. *Healing Yourself: A Step by Step Program for Better Health Through Imagery.* New York: Wahlen and Co., 1987.

Shames, K. *Creative Imagery in Nursing.* Albany, NY: Delmar Publishers, 1996.

Singer, J. *Boundaries of the Soul: The Practice of Jung's Psychology.* New York: Anchor Books, 1972.

9 | THE TRANSPERSONAL PERSPECTIVE

The concept of healing through the human energy field is a powerful tool for resolving deep psychological wounds. The therapeutic relationship allows for blocked energy to be released from the multidimensional field (described in Chapter 7). When this occurs, the client often spontaneously connects with some deeper part of herself such as enhanced creativity and the spiritual dimension. In our experience, energetic approaches potentiate or activate latent spirituality dormant in the client. The work we have described is not a replacement for an active spiritual practice, but instead serves as a catalyst for questioning major issues such as life's purpose and meaning. As clients learn to nourish their own beings they awaken the inner self (the soul) with positive regard, empathy, authenticity, and a sense of hope.

Our goal in this chapter is to explore these concepts further and to demonstrate how the transpersonal perspective enhances the effectiveness of all healing work. Although we focus on client needs, this discussion will also have direct application to the reader. The basic understanding that all healing is ultimately self-healing implies that the therapist works from his own expanded energy field to facilitate balance in the client.

THE SHIFT TO THE INNER WORLD

For most of us, life demands an orientation toward the external world. Our environment, our relationships, unrelenting advertising, and driving from place to place require an alert state of attention to things outside of ourselves. When the external world overwhelms us, or our coping mechanisms fail, we each break down in the part of the human energy field that is most vulnerable.

For some clients, the area of breakdown may be in the specific organ or physiological function that is weakest because of heredity or stress experiences. For others, the emotional field may become stressed, resulting in a constricting emotional pattern such as despair. Distorted thought patterns can emerge, causing neurosis that encompasses more and more of the person's life until she cannot function effectively. Underlying all these dilemmas is a pervasive spiritual disease, a sense of emptiness and discontent. Illness is seen by many depth psychologies as loss of meaning or loss of one's soul (Moore, 1994; Elkins, 1995). For many persons, this sense of emptiness and loss is experienced as a lack of connection to anything greater than the personal self or to one's physically limiting conditions.

Fortunately, physical, emotional, or mental distresses are great motivators. Within every life crisis lies the potential for the individual soul to seek something greater, something which transcends the details of daily life. This hunger, called the "divine discontent" by many sages, is actually the soul's search for wholeness in a disastrously fragmented exterior world.

It is no accident that as our clients release blocked material from the energy field they connect with deeper, more expanded parts of themselves. Insights may be expressed with words such as "Aha, now I see a bigger picture," or with the thought, "My life events make sense in a way I had not considered before." The client's self-awareness and active consciousness allow excessive identification with horrifying past experiences to decrease. It is not that they forget the experience, but rather that it no longer has the overarching emotional pull that it once had. This freeing from emotional bondage leads the client to naturally pursue larger questions such as "What is my real purpose?" and "What is most important to me?" These questions direct the search deeper into the self, where clients begin to connect with a much larger reality, their expanded consciousness, the higher Self, with the capital "S" as described by Jung (1971).

There is now a language that allows us to address emerging individual spirituality without limiting ourselves to bland, neutral phrases or to verbiage that may conflict with the client's religious affiliation. This is the language of *transpersonal psychology*, a growing force in mainstream psychology that builds on the pioneering work of Carl Gustav Jung and Abraham Maslow. Transpersonal psychology enhances the understanding of human nature beyond the realms of traditional psychology by exploring the psyche in relation to the Collective Unconscious, the higher Self, and its quest for spiritual awareness.

Unfolding spirituality is like a budding flower with the potential for exquisite expression of inner beauty. It can be trampled underfoot with the merest hint of judgment or inappropriate wording. Often, as clients experience integration with their expanded energy fields, they report feelings of oneness, a sense of being deeply loved, or even the sensation of a caring presence that is known from their religious backgrounds such as Mary or the Buddha. In attempts to share their inner world, they often say, "You'll never believe this," or show hesitancy about discussing the interior experiences that are new or unusual to them. When this happens in classrooms or individual therapy settings, the helper must step with the gentlest caution and respect.

When we speak of the *spiritual* dimension we are addressing the personal quest for wholeness through aligning with forces that are greater and beyond one's limited ego self. Differentiated from religion, spirituality is very individualistic, a unique reflection of the person's inner search for meaning. While religious groups foster social and external demonstrations of a belief, the spiritual is internal and infinitely creative in its expression. Within religious traditions there is an underlying principle of connecting to a Higher Power or a Supreme Being. This is called the *"perennial philosophy"* by leading transpersonal theorist Ken Wilber (1996) and is a universal concept held in all major spiritual traditions.

Currently, the perennial philosophy and its unique manifestation in individual spirituality is discussed extensively in the transpersonal psychology literature. We might recall that the word *transpersonal* literally means beyond or through the personal. The growing field of transpersonal psychology is a rich resource for the study of the interconnection between spirituality and psychology and adds valuable understanding to the energy-oriented psychotherapy of our discussion.

THE TRANSPERSONAL AS THE
FOURTH FORCE IN PSYCHOLOGY

Jung's exploration into the workings of the human psyche led him beyond the idea that repressed personal material is held in the unconscious past of the mind. He sensed that our dreams, images, and archetypes (discussed in Chapter 8) represent a much deeper and more creative aspect of the human subconscious. And beyond what he defined as the collective human consciousness, Jung explored our greater quest for the unknown, the mystery of our existence, and the meaning of our individual lives. "A basic principle of Jung's approach to religion is that the spiritual element is an organic part of the psyche. It is the source of man's search for meaning, and it is that element which lifts man above his concern for merely keeping his species alive . . ." (Singer, 1973, p. 384). As we connect with this innate wisdom, we move beyond the personal ego self to a wider dimension; the transpersonal, or the Self.

In the United States, a leading light for exploration of the transpersonal was the psychologist Abraham Maslow. Initially, he studied the intuitive flashes of insight and awareness that spontaneously came to some of his patients as they struggled for problem resolution. He called these "*peak experiences*" and helped to move the field of psychology beyond addressing emotional pathology to considering the characteristics and qualities of the emotionally healthy person. Maslow opened the door to the study of emotional wellness and the kind of lifestyles that make someone a "peaker." The human potential movement of the 1970s and the Association of Humanistic Psychology had their origins in Maslow's lifework (Cleary and Shapiro, 1995).

Toward the end of his life, however, after a near-death experience from a heart attack, Maslow began to rethink his work with peak experiences, and developed the less familiar concept of the "*plateau experience*" (Cleary and Shapiro, p. 3–5). This is characterized in the following way by Hoffman, a major Maslow biographer:

> [It is] a serene and calm, rather than intensely emotional, response to what we experience as miraculous

or awesome. The high plateau always has a noetic and cognitive element, unlike the peak experience, which can be merely emotional; it is also far more volitional than the peak experience; for example, a mother who sits quietly gazing at her baby playing on the floor beside her (Hoffman, 1988, p. 340).

The plateau, then, might be considered an evolutionary stage in which the individual matures in spiritual awareness. It is more sustained than the intense "peak" and becomes the basis of a lifestyle attuned to spiritual development. Serenity, with a sense of sustained self-transcendence, is the distinctive feature of the plateau experience. Achieving this higher state of consciousness would require time, work, discipline, study, and commitment in Maslow's view. The important distinction is in the individual's evolution from brief flashes of insight to an abiding sense of light, guidance, meaning, and purpose.

In his last two years, which he called the *"post-mortem life,"* Maslow envisioned a new force in psychology. He stated, "I consider Humanistic Third Force psychology to be transitional, a preparation for a still 'higher' Fourth Psychology, transpersonal, transhuman, centered in the cosmos rather than in human needs and interest, going beyond humanness, identity, self-actualization, and the like" (Maslow, 1968, p. iii). In collaboration with Anthony Sutich and Stanislav Grof, he helped to found the Association for Transpersonal Psychology which recently celebrated its 25-year anniversary.

The Association, with over 40,000 members worldwide, has inspired an entire new format for speaking about the farther reaches of human nature. The spiritual dimension is understood as a natural evolution toward wholeness. Jung called this deepening mature spirituality the *path of individuation.* It may be expressed by the individual through specific religious or meditative practices. It may be reflected by holding a deeply personal connection to the greater universe, the forces of nature, or a sense of inner joy. Each person's distinctive way of reaching to the numinous is honored and respected. Everyone's path is considered valid, from prayer to meditation and contemplation, in orienting toward the deeper Self. In fact, these methods for connecting to something larger than the personal can vary enormously, ranging from the many forms of yoga and centering to repeated, daily rituals. All are considered meaningful, each reflecting yet another creative aspect of our divine potential.

"Exploring the inner world of soul calls for discernment and discrimination, knowing when to confront, when to avoid, and how to transform whatever appears threatening" (Vaughan, 1995, p. 6). Thus writes leading transpersonal psychologist Frances Vaughan in describing aspects of her current psychotherapy practice. Many of today's clients come to psychotherapy with the intent of finding spiritual healing, recognizing their intense need for inner meaning to counteract the loss of soul. Some of the inner work readily moves into discovering further realms of the mind, dream images, symbols of the active imagination, and material that seems to come from other dimensions or the collective unconscious.

Most important in Vaughan's view is ". . . to reinforce the ability to reclaim and heal the soul rather than to reinforce beliefs that are debilitating and damaging" (Vaughan, 1995, p. 4). Addictions, for example, carry a compelling sense of powerlessness with them. This is true whether it be addiction to chemical substances or to compulsive, repetitious behavior patterns. A crisis in the client's personal life becomes an opportunity for paying attention to the soul, and with it, to discover the true Self.

Recovery in all dimensions, then, is the path of self-discovery, reconnecting with the lost aspects, and reclaiming one's spiritual nature. Nowadays, only the most limited of therapies attends to mere problem-solving. More and more counselors recognize that addressing the confusion about inner direction and purpose, the loss of soul, is an essential part of any lasting, meaningful therapy.

THE TRANSPERSONAL DIMENSION IN ENERGY-ORIENTED HEALING

When energetic techniques are applied in psychotherapy, the client often experiences a rapid shift to increased inner awareness. This reorientation to a more internal state of consciousness is a natural result of the embodied presence of caring that emanates from the intentional field of the healer. Beyond the obvious potential for quick rapport, the actual movements of the therapist's hands in the client's energy field enhance relaxation and release of stressors. In traditional "talk therapies," ten or more sessions might be needed to establish a similar sense of trust and inner peacefulness.

Each dimension of the field has an effect on the other layers. The further out in the field the energetic intervention is made, the more pervasive the effect. For example, if we focus on emotional release work, we may impact both the emotions and the physical body. However, if we are able to reach the transpersonal, spiritual dimension, we may effect changes in the mental, emotional, and physical realms as well.

A transformative change is characterized by a major shift in perspective that allows the client a new way of viewing life events or his specific crisis. The client literally needs to move out further to gain an expanded point of view and new insights when confronting a complex problem. Along with this expanded, transpersonal perspective, the client may also understand that there is basic good will in the Universe. Faith and trust in something greater than the material world can grow. Life is seen as more worthwhile when opening to the wider Self: the identified crisis is part of a larger picture. From this point of view, then, the present problem may be seen as less devastating, and come to be appreciated as teaching and an opportunity for learning. The client gains a sense of sacredness, unity, and wholeness that can permeate his entire life.

Creativity is another outcome of this larger window of perception. For the artist, the synthesis of seeming opposites opens new doors to self-expression. For the troubled person, the possibility of looking at dualities and their reconciliation allows new freedom of thought. This includes work with the shadow side and bringing it into awareness.

As we describe the specific case examples in succeeding chapters, the transpersonal is considered to be an integral part of the healing process. Change in individual lives comes through expanded consciousness that reaches to the higher Self and its supportive Source. The result becomes manifest in greater creativity and flexibility, a far cry from merely developing coping skills. The individual feels more connected, both to his own internal resources, and to the wisdom that reaches beyond the ego self to the transpersonal dimension.

NURTURING THE TRANSPERSONAL ASPECT IN PRACTICAL WAYS

In addition to psychotherapeutic considerations, we want to recommend practical ways that all of us, healers and healees alike, can connect with the transpersonal perspective. The "high plateau" that Maslow described is maintained and nurtured through daily intent and purposeful activity. The following are practical suggestions that can enrich therapeutic interchanges to encompass the spiritual spectrum of the human energy field.

Conscious Movement Beyond the Personal, Temporal Self

Much of our identity on a day-to-day basis is concerned with what we do and have. Statements such as "I am a doctor, a psychologist, a nurse, a mother, an entrepreneur" describe activity, levels of academic achievement, and current success succinctly. "I am a survivor of World War II in Berlin, of suicide, of a dysfunctional family, of incest, of near-death experiences" name a client's past problems and emotional work areas, albeit in a rather constricted way. Similarly, "I am an alcoholic, an approval junkie, an overeater, an addict to perfection," or the like may be descriptions of some clients' current addictive patterns and serve as a temporary point of self-identity.

In 12-step programs, the admission of one's debilitating condition (step 1) is immediately followed by a transpersonal statement (step 2). "Admitted the we were powerless over [the substance or condition] . . . that our lives have become unmanageable . . . came to believe that a power greater than ourselves could restore us to sanity" (Alcoholics Anonymous, 1978). We need to move beyond describing ourselves in terms of activity, troubled past, or addictive patterns to statements of who we are in relation to a larger framework. Thus, "I am a seeker for truth" or "I am a beloved child of Creative Mind" captures our transpersonal essence. The heart of our being, who we really are, needs to be valued in speech and action.

One suggestion is to make it a practice to state to yourself who you are in relation to the cosmos at least once a day. It is fun and very enlightening to think of one sentence by which you would like to be remembered in history, or to write down the message you want placed on your tombstone.

Make it a habit to follow every day-to-day activity with an acknowledgment of ways the action nurtured your spirit. For example, "I pulled weeds to get it over with and tidy up the yard" is quite different from being really present in the moment and essence of the task. As we open to the experience and its transpersonal aspect, we might say "I pulled weeds for two hours this morning and with it I connected to great Mother Earth. I became one with the will to live that is reflected in even the most humble plant shoving its life force through a rock crevice."

The Practice of Continual Centering

Because centering is an integral part of all healing work, it is a useful practice before any new beginning. Getting into the car, visiting someone, making a telephone call, going into an unknown office, setting out and returning—every life activity becomes deeper, fuller, and richer if we set our intent, and acknowledge the support of a friendly, teaching Universe. With practice we may acquire a sense of being centered more and more automatically so that this heightened awareness is available in times of crisis.

Working with others becomes more intuitive and more genuine when we are centered. As the ego self steps aside, our fuller awareness can emerge and things begin to flow. In the helping professions it is very powerful to stand back for a moment and let ideas and images come to us. Again, we gain a new perspective as we move higher, out of the defined problem, to transpersonal awareness.

Exploring All Challenges from the Transpersonal Perspective

The helping professional, whether client or therapist, has a tremendous imperative to attend to his transpersonal development. How else could one address a clients' deepest fears without sinking into one's own unresolved material? Death and dismemberment, for example, seem to be pervasive in the collective human consciousness. For many, this is the ultimate fear that underlies *angst*, anxiety, neurosis, and "the worried well." We need a framework that goes beyond the drama of the worst imaginable event.

Addressing our own fears of death may send us on a quest of reading and insight. We might ask from a transpersonal viewpoint, "Who or what really dies?" From what we have learned of near-death experiences (Moody, 1975; Atwater, 1988, p. 6), physical death is a transition to another form of life, somewhat akin to taking off a tight shoe. Consciousness continues in some form, similar to the way we awaken from a frightening dream. Working with client fears directly while the therapist maintains his centered field supports expansion of the client's resources toward the transpersonal dimension.

Seeking the Synthesis in Duality

Psychospiritual integration requires that we embrace our seemingly contradictory natures (Small, 1994, p. 149). Sometimes our humanness is all-absorbing, as in intense grief; sometimes we catch sight of our divine nature and experience a sense of life creating itself anew after loss. The more we seek light and understanding the more we tap into dark and unknown aspects of ourselves.

Awareness of the shadow within is an eminently useful way of connecting with the higher dimensions of Self. A simple exercise is to make a list of all the qualities within yourself that you currently like and appreciate. Then make a second list of the down-side, the disliked aspect of that quality.

When nurse Jennifer made her list of positive attributes, she quickly came up with "organized, ability to plan ahead, and pleasant." With each quality she then paired an opposing aspect: organized paired with being compulsive; planning ahead was associated with worrying about the future; being pleasant related to being gullible or overly adaptive. Quickly Jennifer had a picture of her personal shadow side as gullible, worrisome, and somewhat compulsive. These were the very qualities she most disliked in others and that were least well understood by her.

To access the transpersonal dimension we reach higher, to the integration point of these seeming opposites. We might ask "What divine quality is reflected in being both organized and compulsive?" We come up with answers that exemplify positive attributes such as the idea that being both organized and compulsive is connected to seeking out the orderliness of the Universe. Thus, we can see how both the positive and negative manifestations of the personality are reflections of the soul's seeking of wholeness by aligning with divine order or Good Orderly Direction (GOD).

Seen from this perspective, nothing is lost as we expand our consciousness. Rather, we become more balanced as we look at temporarily distorted patterns such as Jennifer's compulsivity and worry. Recognizing the underlying intent frees us from focusing on what is wrong, on pathology or dysfunction, and directs us toward looking at our potential for growth. Like Jennifer, the work cut out for us is to learn to trust the cosmos without personal jeopardy or foolhardiness, being neither too gullible nor too adaptive. We can then enfold the seeming paradox of being secure in the certainty of life's uncertainty.

Opening to Guidance and/or Higher Direction

Remaining receptive to the mystery of our lives may call for a whole new set of values. Our central focus shifts from "having" or "doing" to "being." No lesser person than Mikhail Gorbachev, former President of the Soviet Union, tells us that current political structures, socialism, and capitalism no longer work. The all-encompassing issues of planetary pollution and unlimited consumerism require a massive shift to new values, those in which spirit is primary. He states "It is time for every individual, nation and state to rethink its place and role in world affairs. We need an intellectual breakthrough into a new dimension where the human spirit is paramount" (Gorbachev, 1995, p. 12).

How will these new values, based on the transpersonal dimension, become actualized? Certainly, there must be respect for our natural environment and ecology in as yet unprecedented ways. Appreciation of diversity, both within the human family and all species, is essential. We can no longer afford to see one group as more privileged than another or claim that ours is the most correct way of thinking.

Opening to the higher will is a daily practice of asking how we can best serve or assist others and step out of the quagmire of human conflicts. The following exercise is an example of a path to engage the transpersonal perspective in moving to higher ground.

Exercise: Bringing the Transpersonal into Conflict Situations

1. After relaxing the body in a comfortable position and taking several deep breaths, allow yourself to see a person with whom you currently have a conflict. See and sense the person's presence in front of you.

2. Note which energy center in you is most effected by this conflict. Note the emotion that the image of the person engenders in you.

3. Comfort the emotion of the energy center with full expression of the feeling. For example, "I am now aware of a sensation of fear involving my root chakra." Express the feeling in a safe, active way. Then, follow with an appropriate affirmation. Fear related to the first chakra can be addressed with "This too is temporary . . . My security rests in my connection with Higher Power . . . I sense my boundaries and my energy field . . . Nothing can disturb my connection with my Source unless I so choose."

4. Think of a being whose essence embodies a strong spiritual resource for you such as Mary, Kwan Yin, Buddha, Jesus, Bach, Einstein, or Nightingale. Allow yourself to lift beyond your energy field and the conflicted situation and look at it through the eyes of this higher being. What would this person say or think? What is a sensible next step from this perspective? Shall I let it go, do personal work, confront the person, or express it creatively?

5. As part of your healing ritual, write down what you received from connecting to your resource: light a candle, write a new agreement, smell a flower, do a dance, or release something to the wind. Do whatever symbolizes your next action in relation to the conflict. Remember that great art, music, and literature (in fact all creativity) comes out of the depths of human emotion which has been transformed by connecting to the transcendent.

6. Imagine taking your expanded awareness with you as you meet the person or go to the situation. Notice the change in you as you feel the support of the caring entity with whom you connected. Gently return to full awareness with appreciation of your many resources and strengths.

The reader undoubtedly has noted how the imagery of guidance (given in the previous chapter) is combined with an understanding of the energy centers and the transpersonal perspective in this exercise. These combinations are open to us in infinite variety as we employ an energetic perspective. Work with the human energy field which considers all aspects of the client and is, by its very nature, transpersonal and transformative.

The following case example shows how a series of energetic interventions led the client, Diana, to new integration. This was characterized by direct knowledge of herself, not just thinking or feeling, but the lived experience of her higher Self.

Diana's Story: Transpersonal Integration Through Energy Healing

Diana was a medical student who had just completed her residency. She had been under the care of a physician for an autoimmune thyroid disease and experienced constant shoulder aches and pain. After many long years, she had accomplished much outwardly, but was often drained and tired inwardly. She stated "I need to learn to work with others without depleting my own energy."

On assessment, her field was fuller in the front than back, with a constriction around the shoulders and abdominal area. Her chakras were open, though sluggish, with less flow in the throat and brow areas and no movement around the crown. This suggested a constriction in the center for creative expression (throat center and related thyroid gland) resulting in a diminished capacity to see clearly (brow center), and a blockage preventing connection to her higher guidance (crown center).

Energetic maneuvers were provided to help make more energy available to the entire field through modulation of energy to stabilize and fill the areas around the three upper chakras. She experienced some muscle twitches throughout the session, suggesting a release of blocked energy. Near the end of the first session, there were deep stuttering breaths with expressions of pent-up emotions.

Afterward, she felt much better physically and shared her insights. She likened her life to "feeling really hungry, but not knowing where to get food." Lack of physical intimacy with her husband for several years was one source of this hunger. She also expressed a desire to maintain a sense of vibrancy and vitality through self-care.

Several weeks later, there were significant shifts. She made an agreement to allow herself to feel loneliness rather than to deny it, and to acknowledge lack of fulfillment in the marriage. Assessment on the fourth session revealed that most chakras were open with energy flowing. During the session, Diana experienced a vision of her aunt who had died of breast cancer at age thirty-five, the same age as Diana was at the time of therapy. She felt her aunt had the same sadness that she did, and that her physical problems began around the same time. She realized she did not want to die young from the same empty, hungry feeling.

Diana began taking definite steps toward her own recovery. She started to write in her journal, which opened wide the floodgates of stored emotions. Energetic techniques used by the therapist throughout this time included opening meditations to connect energetically with Diana, the clearing of disturbed areas in the energy field, and modulation of energy over diminished chakras. There were many deep sighs during this work with occasional twitches. At the conclusion of these sessions, Diana commented "I feel I was rocked . . . very pleasant . . . and straightened out."

After one session, Diana drove to all the local places that had symbolic meaning in her life: she traveled in a full circle from her current community to the places where she grew up, visited special sites, and relived past memories. During this drive, Diana had an experience of helping a child who had gotten stuck in mud. She felt this was a symbolic representation of the emotional situation with which she was struggling.

Several sessions later, many changes were evident. She communicated more effectively with her husband, and he was beginning to respond. She felt secure in asking for what she wanted and in setting appropriate limits with the others who made demands of her time. She was giving more to herself, and asking for more. She had increased energy and felt supported by hiring someone to help with the household. She met the challenge of taking her medical boards with a beautiful serene countenance, and even built in a day of healing afterwards, which she spent all by herself in nature. Within a few months, Diana was largely in control of herself and her life, a shining example of transformation.

These are her words about her process:

"When I first came, I knew about the self-care stuff, but I couldn't seem to do it for me. In reconnecting with many parts of myself, I have discovered the value of self-nurturing. In fact, I am finally integrating some old parts of myself that I was unable to know before.

"The energy healing put me in a frame of mind where I could tap into a place where I'm totally accepted for who I am, completely loved . . . It instilled in me that place that babies know, where one feels completely attached and bonded, and adored. I always *believed* in God but then I *felt* His presence (italics ours).

"I had never experienced that unconditional acceptance. I had met with some of that from strangers, but it was more difficult to get from family. However, that pattern is changing as well. My mother gave me a birthday cake last week with a butterfly on it; even she got the symbol for my transformation right! I'm feeling truly seen for the first time.

"There has been a total reconnection to big Self. I needed that on the physical level as well as the emotional level. I've been in therapy for many years, but from the moment you touched my feet, it was extremely healing.

"I was hungry until the moment I came in here; from that moment on, I've felt full. It's like being in the midst of a huge circle; wherever I go, I feel protected and safe."

SUMMARY

Working with the human energy field addresses all dimensions including, ultimately, the transpersonal, intuitive, and spiritual. Of course, the specific images and wording for the transpersonal arise from the client, and the wise therapist moves creatively and flexibly to maximize the client's subjective, interior experience. At its finest, energy healing does not ignore the client's physical issues, emotions, or belief patterns but instead faces them and permits expansion of the psyche beyond its temporal dilemmas. With this comes a reorientation of past events, or a reordering of the current crisis, a sense of empowerment as the energy field is experienced in its new balance and harmony.

In the following chapters we explore how full spectrum healing within the transpersonal perspective addresses specific emotional problems. It important to remember that each individual energy field is one aspect of a much greater entity, the Universal Energy Field, just as each facet of a diamond reflects the larger, more radiant whole. With this in mind, both client and therapist can move beyond the personal ego to boundless consciousness and creative potentials.

REFERENCES

Alcoholics Anonymous. *The Big Book.* New York, NY: AA World Services, 1978.

Atwater, P.M.H. *Coming Back to Life.* New York, NY: Ballantine Books. 1988.

Cleary, T.S., and Shapiro, S.I. "The Plateau Experience and the Post-Mortem Life: Abraham H. Maslow's Unfinished Theory.' *Journal of Transpersonal Psychology* Vol. 27:1, 1995. p. 1–24.

Elkins, D. N. "Psychotherapy and spirituality: Toward a theory of the soul." *Journal of Humanistic Psychology* 1995, Vol. 35:2 p. 78–96.

Gorbachev, M. "Developing New Values" quoted in *Noetic Science Review.* Autumn, 1995, p. 12–13.

Gorbachev. M. *The Search for a New Beginning*. San Francisco: Harper, 1995.

Hoffman, E. *The Right to be Human: A Biography of Abraham Maslow*. Los Angeles, CA: Tarcher, 1988.

Jung, C. G. *The Portable Jung*. Ed. by J. Campbell. New York, NY: Penguin Books, 1971.

Maslow, A.H. *Toward a Psychology of Being*. (2nd ed.) New York, NY: Van Nostrand/Reinhold. 1968.

Moody, R. A. *Life After Life*, Covington, GA: Mockingbird Books, 1975.

Moore, T. *Care of the Soul*. New York, NY: HarperPerennial, 1994.

Singer, J. *Boundaries of the Soul*. Garden City, NY: Anchor Press, 1973.

Small, J. *Embodying Spirit: Coming Alive with Meaning and Purpose*. New York, NY: HarperCollins, 1994.

Vaughan, F. "Shadows of the Sacred: The Power of Imaginal Worlds." *ATP Newsletter* Summer, 1995. p. 3-7.

Wilber, K. *A Brief History of Everything*. Boston, MA: Shambala, 1996.

Section

IV | **ENERGETIC INTERVENTIONS FOR EMOTIONAL DYSFUNCTION**

In this section, we focus on specific psychological issues and ways we approach them energetically. We recall that the basic nature of energy-related work is to assist the client's dynamic field to move to its own harmony and symmetry.

In some cases, this will mean making more energy available for conditions of depletion. Grief, depression, and severe physical illness frequently weaken or diminish the human energy field. Related energetic approaches are described in Chapters 10 and 11. In other cases, harmony needs to be restored by releasing unwanted constrictions or blocks caused by past trauma or abuse. Discussion and client examples of this work are given in Chapter 12. Possible applications of energy healing concepts to relationship counseling and family dynamics are explored in Chapter 13.

10 | ENHANCEMENT OF THE DEPLETED ENERGY FIELD

The most pervasive distortion of the human energy field is depletion. This may be caused by exhaustion, a drop in energy levels before the onset of an illness, the presence of a life-threatening or severe illness, or despair associated with loss. Often, the individual is not even aware of being depleted until there is time to slow down. For example, many participants at our workshop seminars fall asleep during meditations and when they are receiving energy exchanges. After a day or two of resting and rebalancing, they find they are alert and focused while simultaneously feeling relaxed. This sense of vibrant awareness and heightened sensitivity is new and exhilarating. In fact, what they are experiencing as a "high" is actually the state of alert consciousness associated with health and well-being. Many of us carry so much stress and tension in our day-to-day lives that this relaxed/alert state seems like an unusual discovery to us.

Physiologically, this shift toward more balance is understood in terms of interaction between the sympathetic and parasympathetic nervous systems. The overactivation of the sympathetic nervous system gives us stress-related physiological responses (Benson, 1975) exemplified by a state of being "wired" or hyperalert. Balance is restored with the activation of the parasympathetic nervous system and resulting responses such as lower blood pressure, slower heart rate, and peripheral blood vessel dilation. In times of continuous pressure and tension, the body responds with a generalized adaptation syndrome (Selye, 1978) resulting in a compromising of the body's immune defenses, and symptoms such as continuously elevated blood pressure or hyperacidity in the stomach.

At times we may experience a sudden shift when the parasympathetic nervous system becomes activated during a vacation or sleep. The effects of these sudden reversals can be quite remarkable. We are all familiar with the example of pushing ourselves to complete a project or to meet a deadline, and then collapsing into exhaustion and illness during a well-deserved weekend or vacation. We often hear of individuals who drove themselves mercilessly until retirement and died very quickly after reaching their life's goal. Heart attacks, similarly, rarely occur during a hectic workday, but much more frequently at night when the body tries to readjust to its more natural rhythm.

Illness can best be seen as nature's way of getting us to slow down. If we are wise and mindful, we may actually slow down enough to face the underlying issues that are depleting our connection with the limitless supply of energy in the greater universe. Some Eastern teachers of meditation and inner stillness shake their heads at the seeming overactivity that characterizes Western existence. One mystic recently arrived at a new understanding of our busy lives, commenting, "Illness probably *is* the Western form of meditation."

From an emotional perspective, times of rest or introspection often become times of discovering underlying sadness or discontent. Marriages are more likely to experience distress on weekends than when everyone is engaged in activity, even if the activity is not very satisfying or purposeful. The unusual epithet, "The family that drives together, gets mad together" distressingly defines many family outings. To most individuals, quiet time feels like a punishment rather than a gift. The possibility of facing our own emptiness opens up before us like a gaping precipice, and we may rush back to being busy to avoid facing the real pain of the soul.

LOSS AND GRIEF

Since all of us experience loss of some kind throughout our lifetimes, grief and the right to mourn should be well-understood. Not so. Instead, most people seem determined to avoid the possibility of pain through desperate activity until eventually nothing will make it go away. When clients break down and cry, many apologize, as if true feelings might somehow offend. Those moments of truth that manifest in mid-life crisis, in premenstrual symptoms, in work conflicts, or in family arguments are, in fact, the soul knocking on the door of the inner being. They are times to be honored rather than discarded. They may signal the possibility of a new pathway to self-understanding.

Loss of a relationship either by death or attrition is inevitable in every lifetime. Depending on the nature of the attachment and the amount of emotional investment, such loss may require years of mourning and mindful attention. Other losses are also inevitable ranging from loss of a career path, loss of a dream vision or an ideal, to loss of a body function, or loss of libido, the zest for life. Most losses would be manageable if time is taken to respect the feeling, to express grief creatively, and to integrate the learning from the situation. Our society is anything but tolerant of such unfettered time-taking. Hence, many people bury their sadness, telling themselves to "go on" or "get over it" without the necessary working through.

One of the gifts of the energy-oriented approach to emotional healing is the ability to honor whatever emotion surfaces and to allow for its natural expression. Mourning a loss requires unencumbered caring and consistent nurturing, a quality of empathy and warmth beyond words. All of these are available with the energy work. The focused and intentional field of the healer provides a safe, caring place for the client. Words are not needed for the client to receive energy healing. And, as most of us recognize, deep grief is truly nonverbal. Once the emotion is fully recognized and expressed, the psyche can begin to replenish itself.

Another characteristic of grief is its cyclical, seemingly repetitive nature. Living through the stages of grief, as identified by Elizabeth Kuebler-Ross (1979)—denial, anger, bargaining, despair, and acceptance—can move the client to higher levels of resolution and functioning. Most persons, however, do not experience these stages in a discrete sequential fashion; more often than not, there is recycling back through the whole sequence or change from one emotion to the other. If the need for repeated processing is not met, higher levels of resolution and integration are not possible. With energetic approaches we have a direct, noninvasive means of working with a person experiencing loss that can be repeated over long periods of time, allowing the individual to come to gradual resolution.

The inherent nature of the psyche is to heal itself, provided we give it time and nonjudgmental caring. The wise assistant knows when to step aside and when to intervene. Healthy, forward-moving grief work requires the helper to simply stand guard, making sure no self-criticism or premature closure occurs. Unhealthy grieving, where the individual becomes lost in one specific emotion or has a backlog of other problems, requires a much more active role on the part of the helper. We shall explore this as we discuss depression and energy field blockage further on.

Dealing with Intense Grief: Dora's Story

Dora lost her son in a traumatic accident just after he had completed a turbulent adolescence and graduated from high school. Initially, she presented with intense physical symptoms including vomiting, inability to breathe, and sinus pain so deep her teeth felt as if they were all falling out. She was unable to see color and perceived only narrow visual "tunnels" in front of her. When a friend smoothed her energy field for about half an hour at the end of the first day, Dora relaxed, her sinuses opened up, and she was able to see the room around her. After the second time of energy field clearing, a week later, she felt like working in her garden. It seemed as if a film lifted from her eyes when she noticed the colors of the flowers at her feet. As if to underscore the event, a cardinal came to sit on her shoulder (a most unlikely event for those of us who know the elusive cardinal). This seemed like a special greeting from her son who had made a carving of a cardinal for her the previous Christmas. She could not have made that association in her previous state of blurring and numbness.

A week later, after another energy healing session, Dora spontaneously started writing down her thoughts and feelings about her son, the cardinal, the colors, and her garden. She felt his presence and encouragement even during her long, sleepless nights. A month later, she found her son's thesaurus and reread his many letters which she had saved. With the nonverbal nurturing of the monthly energetic interventions, she continued to write, first memories, then poems, then ideas about life on the other side. All of this inner healing work was punctuated by dreams that she incorporated into her journals. Writing became Dora's means of self-expression, her gift as the psyche integrated the complex learning of the grief process. Now, many years later, Dora is a successful writer and poet.

Dora's story exemplifies the possibility of attentive and profound grieving without complications. Much of this was undoubtedly enhanced by Dora's previous therapies, resolution of conflicts, and ability to live more fully in the present. No matter how evolved we are as individuals, grief is an intense, overwhelming experience that requires thoughtful caring. More traditional approaches might have been to give medication for the physical symptoms or to view such an intense emotional state as pathological. Instead, Dora experienced the steady presence of the helper on a regular basis. Sometimes Dora's energy healer commented on feeling like a midwife: "I just allowed Dora to do her work in the context of our relationship." At its best, that is the ultimate healing: to step aside and allow the client's process to unfold. Simple, yes, and very difficult to accomplish, as those of us in the helping professions know.

Addressing Multiple Losses: Rhea's Story

Often, a single loss becomes an avenue for addressing a multitude of related issues. Such was the case with Rhea. Nine months after the death of her husband, she found she could not go to work or even get up out of bed. An attractive woman of 55, she had literally lost all sense of direction in her life. Instead of quickly recovering, as she had expected, the loss was more painful every day until she could not go on, and the flood of tears was incessant.

Initially, her therapist began by encouraging the pent-up sadness to find safe, uncritical expression. Most of the heaviness had been suppressed since her husband's funeral, causing a large backlog of emotional pain. Once the floodgates were opened, Rhea had an intense abreaction with deep, uncontrolled sobbing. The energy work during this time consisted of repeatedly clearing and smoothing the entire field around Rhea. This process allowed for calming at the end of each gut-wrenching therapy hour and provided a safe and comforting container for the intense emotional releasing.

After the first few tearful sessions, Rhea wrote some loving letters to her husband and began imaging him in his new life on the other side. She reread his love notes many times and bought herself flowers, as he had done. She started experiencing a sense of his presence in a comforting way. Gradually, she could speak about him without falling into despair; she even began to admit he had some faults, and laughed about his sense of humor. Their relationship could now be seen as a precious gift without excessive dwelling on the hurt related to his departure. Most importantly, she started to gain self-control and a desire to help others through her work.

The intense opening of the grief work, however, led her to entrust the therapist with other issues. All were losses, albeit of a different kind: her mother had abandoned her, her father was an alcoholic, her first husband abducted their three children to another country for four years, her second husband left her for another woman, and finally, Rhea's daughter had become totally estranged when she reached adulthood.

Each of these issues would, of course, be ample material for in-depth counseling. Within the context of grief work, it was helpful to capitalize on the process that Rhea had worked out for herself. Selecting one issue to work on at a time, Rhea gathered all the memories, images, even notes, about the targeted person and related events. In the safety of the therapeutic setting, she cried, wailed, screamed, and did whatever was needed to allow the emotion its full expression. Her therapist worked with the relaxed state that was available through the energy field clearing, and supported the depleted areas of the field by modulating energy over them. From this relaxed state, Rhea was able to sense her inner wisdom and wholeness. With this internal support, she felt empowered to address the specific person with whom she had a conflict, telling him how she felt, and then releasing the specific individual to continue his own work. Sensing her own energy flow, she also began comforting the inner child or younger self from the past, giving appropriate explanations about what had happened and integrating new insights about the difficult past.

LONG-TERM MOURNING WITH DEPRESSION

A challenge that faces many people because of advances in health care is the long-term decline of a parent, both parents, or a loved one. In the case of Alzheimer's disease or the many neurological disorders associated with aging, we might say that the individual's energies, the very qualities which made him human and lovable, have considerably diminished or totally disappeared. The physical body, however, is still present. Moreover, the body must be cared for even though the personality, the very presence of the loved one, is absent or dramatically altered. This situation creates an unusual and protracted time of loss. The family member, who is frequently also the caregiver, experiences a state of mourning while being in limbo emotionally. The sense of completion that would occur with an actual physical death is missing.

Jerralee's Story

Jerralee came for bereavement counseling concerning grief for her mother. The previous year the mother had been put in a nursing home because of limited self-care capacity and frequent minor strokes. The family expected the mother to die, and all necessary preparations were made. Instead, as her mental condition deteriorated, the mother's physical condition stabilized. Jerralee and her father were left to watch the slow decline of all mental functioning with no definable end in sight. Jerralee was actually mourning her mother's failure to die, a dilemma that would have been less common in prior decades.

Jerralee became increasingly depressed as the months lingered on. She continued to visit her mother on an almost daily basis. When asked about this seemingly excessive visitation schedule, Jerralee said she felt obligated. Her sense of obligation was rooted partly in a strong religious upbringing and partly by being the responsible oldest child. The obligation was underscored by being named after both parents. Now, the sense of duty had become a distortion, a form of emotional self-abuse. The slow, long-term nature of her mother's illness was depleting Jerralee and creating signs of major depression.

The loss of a loved one, while the body is still alive, is an unusual state that is psychologically confusing. There is, in fact, no foreseeable end to the grieving. The pervasive sadness can easily become a state of depression, as was happening with Jerralee. The therapist chose to approach Jerralee with traditional assessment for the severity of the depression. Was there suicidal ideation? Was there impaired physical functioning, sleep or eating disturbance, psychomotor retardation? Was medication indicated from a clinical point of view? Since none of the symptoms were severe enough for medication or hospitalization, a more conservative course of treatment could be used with careful monitoring to notice any worsening of her condition.

In addition, the therapist used energy field assessment and found the entire field depleted, flat, with no bounce or vibrancy. This systemic depletion became the focus of weekly sessions to create more balance and vitality in the field. Initially, the therapist helped make more energy available to the field by imaging a spinning movement through the field, while holding her hands over each of the major joints and chakras (details of this procedure are described at the end of the chapter). By the second session, Jerralee learned how to work with her own energy field daily by connecting the energy centers with each other.

After several months of psychotherapy and work to enhance the energy field, Jerralee began to feel more alive. Anger about the situation with her mother surfaced. Jerralee began to verbalize the unthinkable: God had made a mess of her life. After this realization, Jerralee's despair and sadness gave way to attempts at finding better ways of coping. If God would not fix her life, she decided, then she had better take responsibility. The mother's condition was relatively stable, allowing Jerralee to feel more comfortable about making less frequent visits. Jerralee started going out with her friends and developed more supportive relationships. With the support of the energy healing she also started feeling more connected to her Higher Power. Skills learned years before, when she was in a 12-step program for alcoholism, came back to her. She found going to meetings helpful and connected with old friends.

Jerralee's emotional work was slow and steady. Gradually, changes came: she smiled more, cried less, and began to have a sense of inner well-being despite the unresolved situation with her mother, who continues two years later as before. Jerralee smoothes and balances her mother's energy field on her visits, now held twice a month, to reduce her sense of helplessness. Most important, Jerralee has a sense of empowerment in relation to her own energy field. She does meditations connecting to the chakras daily. She attends classes and is learning actively how to assist others who can respond more fully to her ministrations. Her life has moved from passive watching of her mother's decline into active seeking of emotional and spiritual unfolding.

WORKING WITH DEPRESSION FROM AN ENERGY PERSPECTIVE

Active grief work related to loss is quite different from depression. Emotionally, the mourning of a personal loss can be quite direct and focused. Depression, on the other hand, is often a more pervasive response to numerous losses. Sometimes, the depression can actually be traced to an event, such as incomplete grieving over a death, leading to many suppressed feelings. This may have occurred years prior to the onset of depressive symptoms. At other times, there is no specific event, but rather a state of generalized despair and hopelessness.

Unexpressed anger can also cause severe depression. An enormous amount of emotional energy is required to hold in real and justifiable anger or to deny its presence. The person may become so charged with the burden of resentment and rage that the body and surrounding energy field becomes intensely blocked. Less and less life-supporting energy can flow into the system or outward, causing severe energetic depletion.

In the human energy field, the differences between recent, acute loss and pervasive depression are quite remarkable. Acute grief may cause a flattening of the field with diminished vitality, but this is usually quickly relieved when there is adequate time to express the feeling and facilitate clearing of the heavy emotion from the field. Chronic grief, such as seen in depression, results in a much more sluggish field that is depleted on assessment but responds only very gradually to energetic maneuvers.

More severe depression requiring medication is also amenable to energy healing concepts. The energy work actually enhances the effectiveness of medications. Although we are not certain of the mechanism for this, the increased effectiveness of medication is a well-known effect of energy healing that has been researched and documented in the literature about energy healing (Quinn, 1987; Krieger, 1993). Another effect of working energetically is the resulting sense of personal empowerment. Clients can sense their own energy when they move their bodies, when they pass their hands over the field, or when they feel their own chakras. Above all, the energy work adds no harm, an important consideration when looking at the possibility of medication overdose and addiction.

Tammy's Story

Many reach mid-life with a sense that life has passed them by and that there is little hope of achieving one's goals. Tammy's children had left home, her husband provided well, but she had no sense of purpose in her life. She became increasingly depressed, and despite medication, was often unable to face getting up in the morning. Clearly, this was not the situational kind of depression that would easily lift with antidepressant drugs; the issue of her emptiness and lack of interest in life would require careful, steady attention. Her husband was preoccupied with his work and initially did not wish to recognize Tammy's illness.

Tammy's therapist began by telling her about the principles of energy-related healing. Tammy responded by finding several books on the subject. "I might as well do something," she sighed. Each week she asked more questions about the energy centers. She began exploring the idea of helping herself through the meditation described later in this chapter. The real breakthrough to her apathy, however, occurred when her pet cat was injured in a fight. This gave Tammy an opportunity to try out the energy interventions she had learned and to feel needed. At her garden club meeting the following week, she found she had something interesting to say when she described her pet and the rapid wound healing that followed her gentle maneuvers.

Pursuing this interest in animals, the therapist suggested that Tammy explore volunteer opportunities at the local humane society. Tammy signed up, took the volunteer training and found that there was plenty for her to do. Her life has become fuller and richer as she brings her nurturing talents, long learned in being a mother, to the animals. She has a reason for getting up in the morning, and even her husband is more attentive. She plans to wean herself off the medication gradually in the next six months with the continued support of counseling and energy field balancing.

IDEAS FOR ASSISTING A DEPLETED ENERGY FIELD

Initially, the client may need the therapist's help to facilitate connecting with increased personal vitality and energy. As soon as possible, however, it is best to encourage the client to use energetic techniques herself. The concept of self-empowerment is thereby built into the treatment plan. The other advantage of client participation is resolution of any confusion the client may have about the therapist's seeming external manipulation of the energy field.

The Chakra Meditation Sequence, focusing on the individual energy centers (presented in Chapter 5) is helpful in awakening curiosity and hopefulness in depressed persons. In our experience, it is best to voice-guide the client through the meditation if the client is receptive. This allows the client to become aware of her own responses quickly and to reflect on the sensations, memories, or images that arise while modulating energy over each center of consciousness. Adding affirmations appropriate to the client further enhances the effect.

Another useful energetic idea is that of connecting the energy centers while imaging a spinning, clearing movement. *Chelation* literally means to "claw out" or to "spin out." As a medical technique, chelation is used intravenously to attract free radicals that cause plaque formation, thereby cleansing the blood of patients with coronary artery disease (Chappell, 1995, p. 55–56). In terms of the energy field, chelation is a means of spinning out and cleansing the accumulated debris in the energy field, termed *"clogged auric mucous"* by Rev. Rosalyn Bruyere, author of *Wheels of Light* (personal communication, Nov., 1993).

Chelation of the energy field is a noninvasive but often very effective means of helping with energetic depletion. The depressed client can be encouraged to image a spinning, clearing motion in each of the major joints and chakras, while following the sequence described in the following exercise. This process is adapted from the work of many well-known healers and is variously called the Chakra Connection (Joy, 1979), Chelation (Bruyere, 1987), Full Spectrum Healing (Brennan, 1989), and Full Body Connection (Mentgen in Hover-Kramer, 1996).

This exercise shows how a caring friend or therapist could speak directly to someone in grief or depression to assist increasing the flow of energy in the chakras and related field.

Exercise: Connecting the Energy Centers

1. Ensure you have a quiet environment for 20 minutes and let yourself be comfortable.

2. Set your focus and intent for health and well-being, feeling the support of the limitless resources that are available from your Higher Power.

3. Connect your hands to the nondominant foot and ankle helping to make available warmth and a flow of life-supporting energy.

4. When you feel warmth and a sense of love and peace in the foot, allow your hands to connect with the ankle and knee on the same side.

5. When the lower leg feels "full," let the hands move to connect the knee and hip. Each hold so far might take 1 or 2 minutes.

6. Follow the same process on the dominant side of the body, connecting foot to ankle, ankle to knee, and knee to hip.

7. Now hold both hips and allow the warm flow of your caring and alignment with Source to fill the lower pelvis. When you work with your own body you will know exactly how long to hold each area, and you will also be able to note any emotion that arises as you do this work.

8. Connect the root chakra at the base of the spine and the sacral chakra, letting the lower pelvis fill with light, warmth, and love.

9. Move the hands to connect the sacral and solar plexus centers. This is often an area where one feels very vulnerable and depleted, so you might want to add the image of building a protective energy bubble or shield over this area.

10. Move the hands to connect the solar plexus and heart chakras, again holding as long as needed and sensing the protective layers of the field.

11. The hands and arms are the extensions of the heart center, so they are next in the sequence. With one of the hands, connect the wrists, elbows, and shoulders sequentially as you did earlier with the feet.

12. Return one hand to the heart center and place the other over the throat area, contacting your creative potential for expression.

13. Connect the throat and brow centers, sensing your many intuitive gifts.

14. Let the hands move over the brow and crown to facilitate your sense of higher purpose and meaning.

15. Finally, let one hand rest over the crown and the other reach out to the points above the crown. This can symbolize connecting to the Infinite, the Transpersonal, the Higher Resources.

16. Feel the integration of your body, the chakras, and the related layers of the field affirming your right to be fully alive and present in the world. Write down or share any insights that come to you.

SUMMARY

Thinking in energetic terms gives us a new perspective for working with grief and depression. With these concepts we have integrative, nonverbal, and noninvasive means of working with persons in need. We often sense that something more than talk is required to resolve grief or touch the depths of depression. This work, therefore, can be a resource when we need to reach beyond words and tap into deeper resources to assist those in need.

Since many forms of energy field depletion are associated with physical distress and severe illness, we explore energetic approaches for those issues in the next chapter.

REFERENCES

Benson, H. *The Relaxation Response.* New York, NY: Morrow and Co., 1975, p. 23.

Brennan, B. *Hands of Light.* New York, NY: Bantam Books, 1987, p. 201–233.

Bruyere, R. *Wheels of Light.* Arcadia, CA: Bon Productions, 1989.

Chappell, L.T. "EDTA Chelation Therapy Should be Used More Commonly in the Treatment of Disease." *Alternative Therapies.* May, 1995, Vol 1:2, p. 53–57.

Joy, B. *Joy's Way.* Los Angeles, CA: J.P. Tarcher, 1979, p. 271–275.

Krieger, D. *Accepting Your Power to Heal.* Santa Fe, NM: Bear and Co., 1993.

Kuebler-Ross, E. *On Death and Dying.* New York, NY: Bantam, 1979.

Mentgen, J., in Hover-Kramer, D. *Healing Touch: A Resource for Health Care Professionals.* Albany, NY: Delmar, 1996, p. 105–114.

Quinn, J. "Building a Body of Knowledge: Research on TT," *Journal of Holistic Nursing.* 1987. Vol. 6, p. 37–45.

Selye, H. *The Stress of Life.* New York, NY: New American Library, 1978.

11

WORKING WITH ENERGY FIELD DEPLETION RELATED TO PHYSICAL ILLNESS

Since the affective domain is closely interconnected with the physical, all severe physical illnesses carry the potential for emotional depression. The current understanding of the close interrelationship of body and mind, psyche and soma, is exemplified in the new discipline of psychoneuroimmunology. The body/mind connection forms the foundation of the holistic worldview that gives complementary modalities their entry into mainstream health care settings.

For example, in the case of cancer and AIDS, the suppression of the immune system seems to be closely linked with emotional depression. As the physical symptoms exacerbate, depression deepens; as depression lifts, physical functions improve. Some theorists postulate that mental messages of discouragement and hopelessness actually become translated through the neuropeptides into diminished immune function (Pert, 1986).

Increasingly, medical attention is focusing on other diseases that result in severely compromised immune systems as well. Examples of these disorders are Chronic Fatigue Immune Deficiency Syndrome (CFIDS), Environmental Illness (EI), pervasive metabolic disorders, and the many syndromes that result in chronic, long-term pain. All of these diseases are difficult to treat and have strong emotional components. Many physicians refer their patients for psychiatric assessment and counseling when they have exhausted the usual avenues of medical treatment.

Ultimately, of course, there may be no cure or clear resolution of these long-term, complex conditions. It appears that the more emotional and financial resources patients have, the more likely they are to seek out alternatives and thereby find some relief. In addition, these seekers can at least rest in the comfort of having explored all that is available in our current state of knowledge.

As we look at the model of the interactive layers of the human energy field (described in Chapter 4), we can readily see how working with the field might impact the entire energetic system, including the physical body. Assisting someone to gain new perspectives and work with positive thought patterns can lead to conscious changes in lifestyle. As the person's habits become more intentional, he may feel empowered and capable of dealing with physical dilemmas. As the emotional body is encouraged and supported, the physical may follow with increased immune system functioning and enhanced endorphin production.

In this chapter, we explore our work with clients who sought out integrative practices of psychotherapy because of their psychosomatic illnesses. We will describe how we approached the depleted energy field and the results that came from the combination of energy healing with psychotherapy.

One might argue forever as to the etiology of the clients' distress. We could ask questions such as "Did the somatic component originate from unresolved past conflicts?" "Was the depression present before the illness?" Or "Did the illness lead to depression?" In other words, which was first? Unfortunately, these lines of pursuit would not give us solutions. The person in pain would still be in pain even if we arrived at the most definitive diagnostic answers.

It seems that a flexible, fluid approach, including various options and resources, is most effective with these clients. In many cases, we simply worked directly with the clients' energy fields and chakras to help them release blocked emotional tension. As the client learned to expand beyond the constricting emotion, he began to access new ways of approaching his life. The art of therapy is in guiding the client to his own solutions and finding the unique combination that will work for him.

ACUTE PHYSICAL AND EMOTIONAL CRISIS

In many individuals, emotional distress is first noticed when physical symptoms set in. Because of this, many persons do not seek therapy for their emotions until the physical body demonstrates frequent breakdowns, signifying an impaired immune system, or when recovery from an illness is unusually slow. Typically, clients will say "I just can't seem to shake this thing; I wonder if there is some other reason." The earlier the holistic interventions begin, the better the prognosis for resolution. Thus, when we see someone with acute physical and emotional distress, like Darla, there is a good opportunity for assisting with deep and far-reaching changes.

Darla's Story

Darla was a graceful woman in her early seventies who had made a name for herself as a university professor teaching others how to use their creativity. She was also the survivor of a life-threatening illness, and provided a powerful role model for others.

When she first came to therapy, she had returned from a trip abroad. She was in acute distress with breathing difficulty and was on antibiotic treatment. She also had an auntoimmune metabolic disorder but had stopped her medication for that condition several months earlier because of neglect. In addition to the physical distress, however, there was a sense of urgency, a feeling that something else was going on, although she could not verbalize the reason for this.

All chakras appeared diminished on initial energy field assessment. There was heat and constriction around the heart area. The therapist followed her awareness of the symptom and asked, "What is happening with your heart, Darla? What is causing you tension here?"

Darla's response was an immediate gasp followed by an explosion of emotion. "Yes, I would imagine there's something going on there!" she exclaimed. "My favorite granddaughter has run away, and they found her this morning in the crime-ridden Westside District. She was staying with some druggies!" Darla's face showed her agony and rage. "It's all because of her mother! That girl just won't listen to me. I raised her well, but she's raising her daughter in a way that defies reason. The child has no choice but to run away and look elsewhere for love. I've just become aware that the man the mother is living with was molesting the child. No wonder she ends up with drug dealers." (The therapist made a note, of course, to explore the molest issue before the end of the session and take appropriate legal action, but that is not the main focus of our discussion here.)

As she was speaking, the therapist gently modulated energy over the front and back of the heart center as Darla wheezed and gasped. Eventually, she began to cry and to release huge sobs with moaning sounds. At this time the healer moved the hands over the sacral area since this center is most associated with the release of feelings. After many minutes of expressing her emotions, Darla sat up and smiled. "I guess there really was a lot in there," she commented, noting how much better she felt. Later, at the end of the session, the field was smooth and balanced. Darla promised to take her medication again and to return soon. She was amazed at how powerfully energy was moving through her body, and that she could feel it so clearly.

On the next visit, Darla was physically improved but still felt exhausted. Assessment showed that the energy field was diminished, with all the chakras slightly open except for the crown. After systemic balancing by connecting the energy centers (described in Chapter 10) to help make more energy flow available to the field, the therapist worked specifically with the crown center to assist Darla's connection with her inner guidance. As the work proceeded, Darla relaxed, her breathing became steadier and deeper, and she began to smile slightly. Darla sought out the resource of prayer and asked for guidance in what to do next to help her granddaughter.

In the following session, Darla was in better physical health and more amenable to work on the emotional issues that so plagued her. The teenager had been placed in a private school that was the only alternative to juvenile detention. Over the next few weeks, Darla and her therapist explored Darla's role as family caregiver, and her co-dependency issues in light of the recent family events. She responded readily to hands-on work, which seemed to help her relax as she considered her decisions. Currently, she continues to feel very sad about the entire situation, but she is able to step back more objectively without being overinvolved. She is enjoying life more fully and returned to her own work of helping other professionals with their creativity.

LONG-TERM PAIN

Many clients come to therapy with long-term, intractable pain, having reached the end of all available medical treatments. The idea of a quick solution by means of medication has to give way to more realistic notions. One of these might be to appreciate partial relief and to increase awareness of the stressors that exacerbate the discomfort.

Since there is no effective external objective measurement of internal pain sensation, we begin each energy healing session by asking the client to rate his pain on a scale of one to ten. "Ten" represents the worst pain ever experienced in one's lifetime, and "one" denotes minimal pain sensation. With this simple device we have some means of determining at the end of the session if there has been a change, even to a slight degree. We assist clients in setting realistic goals, modifying the idea of cure to consider gradual, increased self-understanding and self-management as part of their healing. In fact, we attempt to help clients explore the nature of multidimensional healing set forth in this book.

Since we know that energetic approaches help to enhance the action of medication, the client may gradually decrease his use of medication. With less medication blocking the neuroreceptors of the pain-perceiving neurons, the client may actually begin to produce more of his own internal chemical molecules for pain control, known as endorphins (Cousins 1983).

Phil's Story

Phil was referred by a medical doctor for recurrent low back pain. He was also beginning to show signs of depression. Interviews in the first two sessions showed that he was a sixty-year-old widower who deeply missed his wife. In addition, he was burdened with a complicated legal entanglement. He was involved in a zoning dispute that had lasted for several years after a neighbor complained about his converting the garage into a living space for his daughter. She was his only living relative. The neighbor seemed determined to aggravate Phil and had quite literally become "a pain in the ____," where the current physical symptoms were evident.

On the third session, the therapist suggested exploring energy-oriented healing work. Phil responded positively as rapport had already been well established, and he was most eager for some relief of his low back discomfort. Assessment of the energy field showed a closed sacral chakra. The therapist cleared the energy over the sacral area, helping Phil to release the apparent blockage associated with his emotional distress and completed her work with systemic modulation of the field to integrate the work.

Upon completion of this sequence, Phil bolted upright from the table with a Cheshire-cat grin on his face. He then proceeded to talk about what had transpired with great delight. While the sacral area was being cleared, he saw internal images of a parade of women—in fact, all the women he had loved in his life, starting at a very young age—coming to offer him support and pleasant remembrances. This evidently was exactly the medicine he needed as a lonely widower. He shook the therapist's hand vigorously as he departed.

He never came back for further work. Whenever the therapist meets him in the community where she lives, he radiates a big, warm smile. Recently, he grabbed her arm and told her of an unbelievable event that had happened. He had met a woman, someone special to him, and was soon to be married. He laughed with glee as he shared his story of triumph over the internal demons. He was free from pain, and credited the energy healing with his release.

Carol's Story

A woman in her late thirties, Carol came to psychotherapy with both physical and emotional symptoms. She had two young sons and was a single parent. Some months prior, she had visited a dentist who informed her that he wanted to provide a "maintenance process" that he performs regularly. This process, unfortunately, left her with severe repercussions.

Not only was her bite adversely affected, but also her disposition and finances. Evidently, the "evening out" of the teeth upset the balance in her jaw, dislocating her bite. She had already spent $30,000 trying to repair the damage without success. In the midst of this trying experience, she also noticed a decrease of vitality and was diagnosed with a thyroid disorder.

In the initial session, the therapist focused on the physical issues related to the throat energy center. Later, Carol learned about the psychological meaning of the throat chakra. She identified a lifelong pattern of difficulty in speaking out, sharing her inner sense of truth, and expressing her creativity.

Over the next several sessions, the healing work progressed from clearing out the discomfort in the energy field to discussing Carol's mental, emotional, and spiritual issues. Each session included working through her problems for cognitive insights as well as time for energetic maneuvers and specific clearing and modulating of affected areas. Carol was able to share her resentments, release her rage, and grieve over lost time with her family. She decided to look at her whole life in new ways and named her goal "reworking my response system."

She used the energy therapy sessions to clear up old issues and to connect more deeply with her inner resources. She began to release her sense of panic around the physical symptoms through relaxation and visualization. She acknowledged "I have become more spiritual since all this occurred. I'm actually in touch with more love in my life." Later, she reflected "There is a nice feeling that comes with your energy work. It feels like a rosy glow within. . . ."

More and more, Carol's face began to relax and change shape. At the same time, she felt less pain and more joy. Toward the end of the ten-session course of treatment, she said she felt deep inner peace and mental clarity. She has returned several times for what she calls a "tune-up," and sent notes of gratitude to her therapist.

Lenore's Story

For a year and a half, Lenore suffered from severe, debilitating pain in her right hip and leg. Although no official diagnosis was ever made, her symptoms corresponded to what is currently being called Reflex Sympathetic Dystrophy (RSD) in which nerves, skin, blood vessels, and bones of an extremity are affected (Rosenthal and Wortmann, 1991). In Lenore's case, there was racking pain that felt as if her bones were being scraped alternating with intense burning and deep muscle achiness. As one part of the leg calmed down, another part would flare up with intensity. The skin of the entire leg would, at times, be mottled with red blotches or alternately, pale blue from lack of circulation. She actually considered amputation as the only alternative to making her life more bearable. In addition, she had developed severe allergies to all pain medication resulting in many trips to the emergency room for anaphylactic shock.

With the aid of Medicare, she literally went to every available medical and health care practitioner in her community. Her list of rheumatologists, neurologists, orthopedists, internal medicine physicians, physical therapists, herbalists, and others read like a community resource manual. All to no avail. The gnawing pain persisted and she was unable to take any medication for relief.

She met an energy-oriented therapist when she chose to attend a self-help class for seniors. She ran out of the room dramatically after the first hour in fury and tears. "How can I help myself when I can't even center with all this pain?" she raged.

Indeed, self-help in her state was not feasible. There is a misunderstanding in some therapeutic communities that everything can be handled through intellectual means, changing our thinking, or working with self-help principles. If this cannot be accomplished, many clients think they have failed themselves in some way. Lenore had read the metaphysical and mental science literature widely. She blamed herself for all her distress which only added another dimension of self-hate to the pain. Clearing up this misunderstanding became the first issue in therapy.

The journey toward healing was slow and gradual. Lenore's field was depleted, with most energy centers unresponsive at the beginning of every session. With encouragement, Lenore would vent all her frustration of the previous week, causing a turbulence over the solar plexus center. The excessive energy from her vehement explosions seemed to lend some vitality to the field. Her anger may, in fact, have been her unconscious attempt to enliven her energy system.

The therapist used clearing of the entire field to restore balance at each session. Then, she modulated extensively to help make more energy available and facilitate Lenore's connection to Higher Power. In addition, referral to a psychiatrist who understood energy healing was made early to ensure adequate medical supervision. Because of her stomach problems, Lenore took anti-depressants sporadically, but at least the medication was available as a back-up.

Gradually, her sense of humor returned. Several times Lenore just laughed out loud when she dumped her frustrations about not finding a piece of paper or some other trivial matter. Lenore started to see that she did not have to become so riled up every time something went wrong. Instead, she began appreciating her "spunkiness," her ability to feel things intensely. As her sense of self-appreciation and self-control increased, Lenore's pain sensation diminished somewhat. "I still have pain" she stated recently, "but it's no longer the most important thing in my life."

As her self-esteem improved, Lenore began telephone networking to help a group of seniors in her area. Her knowledge of physicians and self-help groups now makes her a valuable resource to her community. She continues with her program of physical therapy, massage, and medical and group support with daily meditations to maintain optimum functioning of the energy centers.

ENVIRONMENTAL ILLNESS

Certain persons seem to loose the capacity to cope with nature's pollens and chemical products in their environments. This can be due to hereditary patterns and environmental stressors. In these individuals the ability to adapt or accommodate seems to shut down entirely. While most of us may have occasional allergies to food additives or carpet dyes, environmentally ill persons are literally allergic to just about everything in their surroundings. Their numbers seem to be increasing steadily as air and chemical pollution become more prevalent. Medical practitioners are hard-pressed to find effective treatments since almost no intervention is tolerated by these individuals (Rogers, 1994).

More adventuresome patients seek out alternative practitioners and psychotherapy in their attempts to find a feasible lifestyle for themselves. Energy-oriented therapy offers an additional complement to medical treatment of such complex illnesses (Hover-Kramer, 1996, p. 172).

Jenny's Story

Jenny suffered from an environmental illness so severe that she could not even imagine leaving home to go to a physician. She called a counseling center, however, to request telephone counseling for the depression that resulted from her extreme sensitivities. Every time she went into surroundings that had been cleaned with chemicals (a new building or a laundromat) she developed severe asthma attacks, hives, and eye irritations. Although Jenny's request for telephone counseling was somewhat unusual, compliance was possible since she had insurance that covered the costs. In the five telephone sessions that followed, Jenny's energy-oriented psychotherapist taught her how to center herself and to relax her body by clearing her own energy field. This approach was in contrast to more usual therapies that might be directed at finding emotional causes of the extreme physical symptoms and seeming agoraphobia. Jenny had previously tried other therapy approaches that encouraged her to vent her feelings, which resulted in an increase of physical symptoms.

After several sessions of practicing her own self-management, Jenny spontaneously noticed the stars outside the window of her desert home and expressed her sense of deep connection with nature. Using the stars as her image of inner peacefulness, she was able to calm her body whenever she smelled laundry soap and other household items. A week later, sensing more self-mastery, she was able to go shopping for the first time in several years.

She stated that life was worth living again; she was no longer limited by her body's excessive responses. She also confided to her therapist that the name Jenny always implied the tedium that was associated with her illnesses. She now wanted to be a joy to herself and others. "How about calling yourself Joy, then?" the therapist suggested. "Me? can I just do that?" she wondered. She paused and then added, "Why not? I'm trying so many new things I can just let myself be a Joy." And it is true: she has more joy and purpose in her life since the short course of therapy.

CHRONIC FATIGUE IMMUNE DEFICIENCY SYNDROME

Chronic Fatigue Immune Deficiency Syndrome (CFIDS) is understood medically as a viral infection that totally depletes the body of its resources, resulting in ten or more identifiable symptoms (CFIDS Chronicle 1994). Typically, before onset, the patient has a very active lifestyle in which little attention is given to the body's need for rest and balance. Instead, the person is used to being very active, "burning the candle at both ends," so to speak, with all the endocrine glands running at their peak. In our culture, these people are often recognized and admired as high achievers who never slow down. After many years of this lifestyle, however, there is literally no ability to "turn off" the mechanism of the highly stressed system until total exhaustion sets in. At that point, similar to the battery of a car that has been left on for a long time, nothing will start; there is almost no life force left.

Recovery from this debilitating condition can take years, or it may never occur. Some of the potential for recovery depends on the extent of the damage, the patients' willingness to learn a new lifestyle, and the body's restorative mechanisms. The emotional frustration of being literally commandeered to change one's entire life pattern is especially difficult for high achievers. Discouragement can turn to depression and bring high suicidal risk.

An holistic approach combining medical supervision, client self-awareness, and emotional support during the long recovery phase is essential. Thus, many CFIDS sufferers seek out psychotherapy to deal with their emotional distress. Finding meaningful tasks that do not strain the physical body is difficult at best and requires daily monitoring.

Paula's Story

Paula was a successful businesswoman, well in charge of herself and the world. She was constantly adding new projects to her already overfull schedule until one day "the flu" kept her in bed. Unfortunately, she could not recover. Months later, she was barely able to do minimal self-care, and visits to a long list of medical specialists gave little promise or hope. She was totally disabled. After two years, she met the criteria for Social Security disability payments, a humbling step down for someone who had been so active, financially successful, and self-reliant.

In her third year of doing practically nothing other than telephone answering, she decided to return to college and get a counseling degree. In her psychology program she learned about the energy therapies. Deciding she had nothing to lose, she sought out a practitioner who combined years of counseling experience with energy healing concepts. Thus, she learned about her chakras and how to keep them open with gentle spins (described at the end of the chapter). In addition, she learned how to boost her energy field with the connecting of the energy centers (described in Chapter 10). She further learned how to relax herself whenever there was stress, to slow down her system, and to prevent further "burnout."

Three months later, Paula was completing her first full semester of school without any increase in her physical symptoms. Her spirits have lifted and she is hopeful. "Who knows, " she mused, "Maybe I'll specialize in counseling others with CFIDS since so little is known about its treatment. I certainly know what I'm talking about."

Exercise: Spinning through the Energy Field

This exercise is especially effective with persons who have very depleted energy fields and severe physical illness. Ideally, the client would move the body, especially the hips, in a clockwise spin as if playing with a "hula hoop." If this is not possible because of physical limitations, strong imagery of spinning the body with vibrant music (Ravel's *Bolero*, Bach's *Brandenburg Concertos*, or lively reggae dance rhythms) can be substituted. The exercise helps to open the energy centers and expand the energy field, resulting in a feeling of vitality.

The therapist voice-guides the client through the sequence in the following manner:

1. As you stand, or imagine standing, make sure your feet are comfortably separated to support the body.

Begin with a smooth clockwise spin from your hips to your right. Allow your awareness to move to the root chakra and literally spin out any congestion in the base of the spine and perineal area, connecting to the comforting support of the earth and affirming your will to live.

2. Gradually, after 1–3 minutes, let your awareness shift to the sacral energy center and imagine spinning through any constricted emotions to clear out the pelvic area. Connect with your ability to feel emotions deeply and give them expression as needed.

3. Next, spin out the solar plexus area while sensing your own power and affirming your ability to communicate and make decisions effectively. If you wish, imagine confronting a difficult person with this sense of personal strength in your body.

4. Move your awareness to the heart center, spinning energy through the mid-chest, activating your capacity to accept others and yourself, and to forgive easily.

5. Your spin may be gentler as you work with the higher centers of the throat, brow, and crown as the energy here is more subtle. Again, affirm the strengths of each center—the will to self-expression, to intuition, and to be in alignment with your highest purpose as you spin your entire body.

6. Complete this 5–10 minute exercise by standing still and allow yourself to feel the flow of energy in your body and sense your beautiful energy field. Imagine moving into your next tasks with this sense of power and purpose. Repeat this exercise several times a day whenever you feel tired and the need to "recharge."

SUMMARY

As we have seen, energetic interventions are appropriate adjuncts for addressing the many illnesses in which physical and emotional dimensions overlap. Because it would be too limiting to suggest single solutions or cures to these complex dilemmas, considering a wide variety of approaches can be exceedingly helpful.

Energetic interventions can easily be adapted to the individual's needs as the case examples show. This kind of work certainly requires ensuring that there is adequate medical supervision. The client's own awareness of his energy field becomes a resource for self-understanding and adapting to the constraints of the illness pattern. Furthermore, complementary approaches offer hope by activating the client's personal sense of power and control. The exercises we have included in Chapters 10 and 11 are enjoyable and allow participants to experience their own energy fields.

In the next chapter, we explore how energy-related concepts are used to assist persons with the complex emotional issues of trauma and abuse.

REFERENCES

____, "A Guide to CFIDS (chronic fatigue and immune deficiency syndrome)" *CFIDS Chronicle*, Winter, 1994, p. 57–58.

Cousins, N. *Anatomy of an Illness*. New York, NY: W.W. Norton and Co., 1979, p. 39–40.

Pert, C. "The wisdom of the receptors, neuropeptides, the emotions and bodymind." *Advances*, 1986, Vol. 3: 3, p. 8–16.

Rogers, S. *The Revised Environmental Illness Syndrome*. Syracuse, NY: Prestige Publishing, 1995.

Rosenthal, A.K., and Wortmann, R.L. "Diagnosis, Pathogenesis, and Management of Reflex Sympathetic Dystrophy Syndrome." *Comprehensive Therapy*, 1991, Vol. 17: 6, p. 46–50.

WORK WITH ENERGY FIELD DISTORTIONS

As we have come to understand, the healthy human energy field is vibrant, smooth, and symmetrical. Many emotional conditions are linked to distortions of the field. These effects may range from turbulence over a chakra that is temporarily affected by situational stress to long-term, established patterns of constriction in one part of the field, and possible overcompensation in another.

We have explored patterns of systemic depletion due to grief, depression, and physical conditions. In this chapter we consider some of the conditions that cause distortions in the flow of energy and ways of dealing with them from an energetic perspective.

ACUTE STRESS REACTIONS

Any trauma, whether emotional or physical, affects the human energy centers and related layers of the field. A simple fall, for example, changes the configuration of the field. Even if there is no discernible physical damage, the area of impact, or its opposite side, is left in a more vulnerable, fragile state. The next time the person has a fall, the resulting injuries can be unusually severe because the protective layers of the field are not at their optimum function.

There are many examples of this phenomenon. Someone who is in shining good health has a severe accident with a minor injury while persons who are already in a deficit seem to suffer ever more with injuries resulting from relatively minor incidents. Similar to the proverbial black cloud, their energy, or more specifically the lack of it, seems to attract further deficits in the form of trouble and discomfort.

Emotional trauma also has a direct impact on the field. Most of us are in such a continual state of being emotionally aroused that we are often less aware of each actual incident, especially if it is minor in nature. It may be helpful for the reader to note the first emotional stressor at the beginning of the day since we are usually most free of emotional debris just after awakening.

Recently, Dorothea went to make her bed after arising and found a very large scorpion on the bedclothes. She backed off in terror, heart pounding, and searched to find suitable means of disposing of the intruder. After that, she noticed weakness in her legs, strong fear (both related to the root chakra), and a need to talk. She called several friends to dissipate the anxiety quickly, to laugh about the incident, as an emotional release, and to establish ways of safeguarding the bed. She completed releasing this comparatively minor trauma by spinning through her energy centers (as described in the previous chapter) to feel grounded, to enhance the energy field, and to open the root center.

Listening to the news in the morning, especially if it is about a subject of personal concern, can affect the emotional field at a time when we are especially vulnerable. The most distressing part of the news is likely to be related to our sense of helplessness and hopelessness. Seeing starving children, maimed soldiers, or persons who are suffering nature's havoc creates an impact on our energy fields that requires some kind of release work. From a psychoenergetic point of view, a conscious activity is needed to shake out the emotional pressure and to rebalance distortions in the field.

In our psychotherapy practices, we create rituals for letting go of fear and anxiety along with helping to bring more balance into the field by using techniques such as the chakra meditation (Chapter 5) or connecting of the energy centers (Chapter 10). Whenever feasible, we encourage action that symbolizes the outgoing, responsive nature of the energy field. Thus, a letter to politicians associated with the situation, a donation of time or money to a favorite cause, a telephone call to the newspaper, or active participation of some form is required for us to remain healthy and balanced in a world that is full of distortions and pain.

Quite literally, we are continually receiving some kind of challenges to our human energies. All of us are suffering from the existential dilemma of living in a difficult, complex world. There seems to be no certainty other than the assurance of constant change. Most of us do not welcome or embrace change, especially of the accelerating, environmentally-destructive kind. Seeing ourselves as spiritual beings having a temporary human experience can be helpful in gaining a more balanced and transpersonal perspective. This may be possible on a day-to-day basis by clearing and energy modulation in relatively healthy individuals. For those who have a backlog of unresolved trauma or other distortions of their field, a much more concerted effort is needed.

CHILDHOOD TRAUMA AND ITS AFTERMATH

Trauma in childhood can cause long-lasting effects in the energy field. We explored the example of Frank in Chapter 7 where a physically and emotionally devastating injury, inflicted at a young age, had a lifelong impact on Frank and his relationship with his brother. The energy field in children is less developed, and according to some intuitive healers, the protective covering over the chakras does not develop until age 7 or later (Brennan, 1987 p. 66). Certainly, common sense would hold that trauma, experienced when we are young, unprotected, and least able to fend for ourselves, can have the most pervasive effects on one's life. Sensing this truth from an energetic concept enhances our understanding and widens treatment options.

Vick's Story

In one of the advanced energy healing classes, Vick volunteered to be the client for the demonstration of back techniques. He was a robust looking special education teacher who experienced constant pain at the left scapula and shoulder. He had visited many body-workers, physicians, and therapists with this problem but basically, it never improved.

The teacher noticed a band of thick, congested energy over both shoulders and the back of the heart center. As she demonstrated the energetic maneuvers to clear out congested matter from the field, she received a mental image of a large hand hitting Vick repeatedly on the left cheek. In her image, Vick's left shoulder moved forward quickly to protect himself from the blows. She said nothing about this in front of the class for reasons of confidentiality. At the end of the demonstration, Vick said he felt about 5 years old and began sobbing. He then composed himself and said he was expressing "tears of gratitude." He reported that the pain had dissipated and he was able to move his shoulder with ease.

When the healer later mentioned privately to Vick that she had experienced a mental picture while working with him, he indicated he was ready to explore further by asking about the image directly. When she told him what she had seen, he cringed. He knew exactly what she was speaking about. His mother, who was a raging alcoholic when he was little, would hit him mercilessly on the left cheek at the slightest provocation. In later years, she went through recovery from addiction, and they were on good terms before she died. Vick did not believe that he still had unresolved trauma from the past because he had consciously forgiven her when she made amends during her final illness.

His energy field pattern of constriction from the battering, however, had remained in spite of his good thoughts. With the trauma apparently stored in his cellular memory and related areas of the energy field, ongoing and specific physical pain had developed. Emotionally, the closed heart chakra resulted in strained relationships, especially with his wife and daughters. The mechanism behind all this was beyond his awareness until he attended the class.

Vick entered therapy ready to work. Fortunately, he found a counselor who understood energy concepts and was able to help him work through his childhood experiences. Despite his initial hesitancy, Vick developed ways of talking directly with his mother, writing her letters, and expressing his anger about the injuries. Just because she was dead and had made amends did not limit his ability to feel deeply about what had happened. Full expression of his anger allowed emotional clearing and gradual release of the blocked energy pattern. After the full expression of the stored emotions, Vick and his mother could realign as friends.

The scapular pain never returned. Vick enjoys his family more fully now, consciously relating to them with an open heart center. His intuitive sense is a growing asset in his work as a special needs teacher.

CHILDHOOD SEXUAL ABUSE

Sexual abuse in early childhood is a therapy issue that is finally being recognized as the far-reaching and pervasive problem that it truly is. When the actual abuse is acknowledged, often after years of suppression, very emotionally charged things can happen. Since the perpetrators of the molestation or incest are often still alive, the molested person deals not only with her own issues, but also must find ways of coping with the perpetrator, including reporting when possible, to prevent further abuse.

It is important to remember that the goal of effective therapy is not confirming or disconfirming the client's experience, but rather helping the client to find paths to living each day more fully. This means helping the client to find ways of participating in life without carrying the tremendous energetic distortion from the molest as the central emotional focus. This working through is needed whether the remembered material is entirely true, partially true, or symbolic in nature.

Abby's Story

Abby had experienced stormy, unsatisfying relationships with all of her sexual partners since her teenage years. Five marriages and numerous affairs, each with addicts of some kind, had left her empty and without job skills or financial security at age fifty. "Something is wrong; my life is a pile of nothing," she said when she came to therapy. She set a goal of getting to know herself better and learning how to live a more satisfying life.

Abby initially gave a vague history about her parental relationships. She was an only child of an older couple. When she described her father she said she was his darling, and together they had won many prizes in ballroom dancing. The father left abruptly with another woman when Abby was 15, never to be heard from again. Abby remembers feeling devastated, "dumped, totally worthless." Because she was very attractive, there were many boyfriends, enabling her to marry and leave home as soon as she was old enough.

Every time she attempted to relax in the counseling sessions, Abby became very uncomfortable. Unpleasant memories were beginning to surface, so she kept busy by talking about daily problems related to her latest man, this time a drug dealer. Assessment of the energy field showed blocked root and sacral energy centers with an overextended solar plexus, the control center. The therapist suggested that Abby do her own centering and chakra meditations daily to help her to feel more in charge. As she relaxed gradually over several weeks, feelings of self-confidence seemed to increase. When she was ready, she shared her terrible secret, which, of course, was not such a great surprise to her therapist: Abby had a sexual relationship with her father from age nine until the time he left.

At first, as she acknowledged the truth, there was an overwhelming sense of betrayal and anger. The therapist supported the abreaction by encouraging Abby to release as much of the pain as possible while assisting with hand movements to clear the heavy, stagnant energy over the sacral chakra.

After the first flood of emotion diminished over several sessions, the therapist suggested that Abby see her father in front of her, at a comfortable distance so she could speak to him. This turned out to be "somewhere near the icy realms of the North Pole." Externalizing the person who had caused her so much pain made it possible to confront him. Throughout this time, the therapist held Abby's hand, by request, to help Abby feel safe in the present, protected from the father's intrusions. With internal imagery, Abby built a "protective bubble," which served as an energetic defense shield that completely surrounded her, further enhancing the sense of security. Abby was able to berate her father for his incredibly selfish, foolish choices and to tell him how her whole life had been beset with sexual confusion because of his actions.

When the therapist suggested visualizing the father getting his own much needed therapy, Abby hesitated at first. Venting her anger was not yet complete, but the possibility of being free to sense her own energy, separate from his, was also intriguing. She worked at her own pace, with the therapist encouraging, but never leading the process, until she was ready. After several anger and release sessions, Abby asked "I wonder how it would feel to be myself, to grow up in a healthy way? I have no idea what that would be like."

At that point the real work of building her own identity began. It was as if Abby needed a whole new past that included loving, nurturing parents who could teach her about sexuality, relationships with men, interactions with other women, and exploring career options. Fortunately, Abby had a flexible imagination and readily experienced these new possibilities like a movie unfolding in front of her. Gradually, over several months, this movie became more internalized, and her own.

When the therapist commented on how creative she was, Abby acknowledged "Yes, I've always been quick on my feet." She began to acknowledge the strengths that had helped her survive the difficult past. She called this quality of survivorship her "Chutzpah," an untranslatable Jewish word for gumption and ingenuity. Gradually, Abby connected to the sense of a Higher Self. She began formulating the goal of attending college and to use her mind in new and challenging ways by studying writing, her secret, lifelong passion.

Somewhere along the line, the current boyfriend became irrelevant, and she started living alone. "Focusing on him was a waste of my precious time; there is so much catching up I need to do," she asserted recently. She continues daily meditation and energy-balancing exercises on her own to maintain her sense of direction. Both Abby and her therapist have noted how the energy-oriented focus helped them to reach core issues without becoming distracted and mired in her upsetting, more external dilemmas.

PATTERNS OF ASYMMETRY

It is customary to think of conditions in the body, such as those related to trauma, as causing distorted patterns in the chakras and layers of the human energy field. However, the opposite could also offer an intriguing description of pattern formation. The field, which is apparently present early after conception, begins to shape emotional and physical configurations that become more evident as the newborn matures. It is as if a formative field exists that creates the structure of the personality and the physical body. Emerging psychological and physiological patterns appear related to the field that provides information forming unique configurations within the individual. This reminds us of the *morphogenetic field* theory advanced by Rupert Sheldrake, who is both a biologist and a creative philosopher (Sheldrake, 1981). The idea of an original field that *creates* the direction and flow of the life force, similar to a riverbed that holds the shape of a stream when rainwater flows, may be a useful analogy.

Thinking in terms of pattern formation may help to understand the severe distortions we see in mental illnesses, especially in those believed to be associated with hereditary and genetic factors. Although the diagnostic considerations of schizophrenia, hyperactivity, bipolar disorder, multiple personality disorder, and dissociative states vary greatly, there are similarities from an energy-oriented point of view. Assessment of persons with these conditions shows a field that is often grossly distorted, deviated, or asymmetrical. Our approach from an energetic perspective, then, is to facilitate repatterning toward symmetry in addition to the other currently known treatment modalities for each category.

Schizophrenia

In schizophrenia, for example, the field is observed to be present mainly above the crown or off to one side of the individual. The colloquialisms of being "beside oneself," or "above it all," aloof and split off, accurately describe the distorted energy pattern of this condition. Energy treatment of schizophrenia would be to help integrate the field, bringing together the disconnected aspects. In early stages of the illness, clearing to balance the energy field can be helpful, but patience and frequent repetition are required. If the patient can connect to a viable sense of his Higher Self and the transpersonal, the schizophrenic episode may actually be part of a breakthrough that can be seen as a form of spiritual emergence (Grof, 1993). In more advanced cases, where there is mental confusion and suspiciousness, working with the field directly may not be possible. However, the helper has much to offer in approaching the person with his own centered, intact field and his clear intent of goodwill.

Hyperactivity

Hyperactivity in children is another condition that suggests hereditary and early patterning distortions. Assessment in hyperactivity shows a wide, irregular energy field with jagged edges. Often, hyperactive children respond to assessment by shaking themselves, similar to a dog after a bath. It is as if they carry too much energy in their aura, more than they can adequately handle. The process of working with hyperactivity is one of learning to modify the excessive energy, bringing it to more manageable proportions. If the parents are available to assist, systemic clearing of the field can be instituted on a daily basis for 5–10 minutes. Repetition reinforces a more harmonious pattern and the energetic imprint of balance in the field. It is as if the child's energy field needs to learn and remember the healthier, calmer pattern. Soothing music, or nature videos, can be used in conjunction with the energetic interventions to further compose the child. Eventually, of course, the child learns self-management of his own energy, beginning with emphatic out-breaths and brushing movements to release the excess energy. It is rewarding to watch children who have been unmanageable in classroom settings experience their own sense of self-mastery with this approach.

Dissociation

Another condition we frequently see in therapy is dissociation. Initially, dissociation is a coping mechanism for severe trauma experienced by someone who has been abused in childhood, as in the examples of Vick or Abby. This mechanism allows the children to survive the trauma without feeling it fully; they become numb and unresponsive to the pain simply by going elsewhere in their imaginations. In adult life, someone who dissociates frequently is literally out of the body mentally and emotionally. This means the person is "not at home" in her field. As a result, the client often bumps into things and accidents occur because there is no way of sensing the physical dimension accurately. Emotionally, the person may be unable to make appropriate responses, even when it is important or life-saving to react. Mentally, others experience the dissociating person as a "space cadet," someone who is ungrounded and off in the clouds or out of touch with reality.

Cindy's Story

Cindy came to her energy therapist after twelve years of other therapies for treatment of childhood abuse, alcoholism, loss of her significant other by murder, and estrangement from her parents.
Throughout the years, she explored the spiritual life extensively. Currently, she meditates daily with a local group. Her goal in therapy was to resolve some of her past issues from an energetic stance since she sensed they still caused distortions in her field.

Energy assessment showed an expanded development of the higher centers and an absence of vibrancy in the lower body. As nothing in the interview suggested physical problems with the pelvis or legs, her therapist asked Cindy about her will to live and related sense of vitality. Cindy explained, "Well, really, I don't want to be alive. I'm not suicidal, I wouldn't do that to my family, but I would be happy to leave my body any time. Come to think of it, I do leave my body a lot; that's why I enjoy meditating so much. I just don't want to be here on the earth."

Again, the energy assessment brought to light a subtle but vitally important condition that the client might not have verbalized so freely for weeks. As it was, the therapist had ample material for consideration, beginning with the very basic issue of dissociation. Since it is not possible to fully release any emotion if one is disconnected from one's feelings, it was essential to build strong bridges to body awareness. Cindy's reluctance to pay attention to the body diminished when the therapist reminded her that the body is the vehicle for spiritual development and linked this understanding to the teachings of her meditation group.

For the first time since early childhood, Cindy learned to know where her feet were located when she was walking. Her therapist instructed her to image her feet as they touched the earth and then to feel the texture of the carpet or ground on which she was walking. Cindy also did the spinning exercise (Chapter 11) and connecting of the energy centers (Chapter 10) as an expansion of her daily meditative practice. With that, she stumbled less often, and there was decreased teasing at her place of work about being from another planet.

With continuous feedback from her therapist and friends, Cindy learned to know when she was angry or in distress, feeling her own emotions more fully. In time, she learned to defend herself when she encountered conflicts and to take appropriate action sooner. She learned to feel alive and vital as a part of her spiritual journey toward wholeness rather than being "in limbo" or only partially in the world. In short, she became more confident and present, enjoying life more fully.

DETOXIFYING FROM SUBSTANCE ABUSE

In the past twenty years, much progress has been made in understanding addictions to chemical substances. Addictions are rightly seen as *dis-ease* of all dimensions, including the physical body's incomplete metabolisms, distorted emotional sensitivities, faulty mental beliefs, and spiritual disconnection. Psychodynamically, we consider the compulsive personality patterns, often coupled with childhood trauma, that lead the individual to retreat into substance abuse as an escape (Black, 1982).

Treatment of this complex disorder is snarled by the body's inability to release the toxic substance to which it has become habituated. In addition, there are usually severe disturbances in the client's social and family relationships, including co-dependency and enabling behaviors. Many addicted persons find themselves shunned even as they try to reintegrate with their jobs and families because of the recurrent nature of the disease. The most effective treatment is the approach of self-management and spiritual reconnecting that is the central focus of 12-step programs.

Energy-related interventions can serve as an additional resource specifically because they also hold the concepts of self-management and transpersonal development as a central focus. In treatment of acute toxicity, clearing of the entire energy field several times a day is beneficial. This unruffling from head to toe should be repeated 15–20 times each session. Anxiety and confusion of the acute stage of treatment can diminish notably with this maneuver. Gradually, the patient learns self-management with breathing releases, centering exercises, and balancing of his own field. As treatment progresses, usually over several years' time, this move to self-responsibility is essential. In addition, the client needs to find ways of sensing his own transpersonal dimension by connecting to his Higher Power in a meaningful way.

Nancy's Story

Multiple addictions are an increasing concern in addiction treatment. Nancy was an example of this. Initially, she numbed herself from the pain of childhood abuse with alcohol. After extensive treatment, she recovered from her habituation, only to find that she had slipped into cocaine addiction. The sequence was similar, with several courses of hospitalization and years of out-patient groupwork. When she found herself stuck in a smoking addiction, with nicotine and marijuana, she decided to try energy healing in addition to her 12-step program.

The spiritual self-help component of the energy work intrigued her and provided another avenue for exploration. Energy assessment on the first visit showed an absence of movement over the second and third chakras and a weak, diminished crown center. Teaching Nancy to gain a sense of personal mastery over her inner demons was crucial. Nancy learned to center herself with peaceful imagery of a waterfall and by listening to calming music. The sense of peacefulness, anchored with breathing, was Nancy's personal connection to the divine through the beauty of nature. She then learned to modulate, or direct, energy from the Universal Energy Field to the second and third chakras.

The daily work of modulating energy became an ideal time to add specific affirmations: "With every breath I now release harmful

smoke from my body . . . With every breath I now increase my resolve to be smoke-free . . . With every breath I now increase my
health and safety . . . With every breath I am adding quality to my
life . . . With every breath I increase my commitment to life."
Because Nancy was a little vain, the therapist suggested including,
"With every breath I am youth-ing myself. With every breath I add
beauty to my entire being."

As Nancy worked with these positive thoughts, she realized how
much garbage there was in her usual mental patterning. The ingestion
of toxic chemicals related to toxic thoughts such as "Men are better;
father knows best; you're not good enough, you can't make it, etc."
She pictured herself clearing out this debris daily with a giant bull-
dozer to make room for incoming light, a pink cloud, and her waterfall. The need to smoke decreased markedly as her anxieties lessened.
Toward the end of six months of energy-oriented healing she said "I
deprived myself and I didn't even know it. It seems as if I'm awakening my soul and noticing the stars and music for the first time."

SUMMARY

As we have explored, distortions in the human energy field
can range from simple aberrations, because of temporary distress, to lifelong patterns of blockage. Some of the most difficult issues in therapy are the ones for which the client can
give no cognitive explanation. The behavior is irrational but
compensates for an imbalance of some kind. Therefore, finding a nonverbal and noninvasive means of exploring the
depths of the psyche opens more doors to self-discovery. The
client's defensiveness is usually minimal because the path to
understanding his own energy is so direct and compelling.

So far we have focused on possibilities for individual
healing with the energy modalities. In the next chapter, we explore the influence of energy awareness for dealing with relationship issues.

REFERENCES

Black, C. *It Will Never Happen to Me!* Denver, CO: M.A.C., 1982.

Brennan, B. *Hands of Light.* New York: Bantam Books, 1987.

Grof. C. *The Thirst for Wholeness.* San Francisco, CA: Harper SF, 1993.

Sheldrake, R. *A New Science of Life: The Hypothesis of Formative Causation.*
    Los Angeles, CA: Tarcher, 1981.

13

ENERGY CONCEPTS FOR HEALING FAMILY RELATIONSHIPS

Anyone who has been involved in human relatedness can sense the power of nonverbal interaction. What allows for communication at subtle levels? What lets us know when we are drawn to someone or repelled, when to reach out, and when to hold back?

The concept of human energy fields gives us a working model for understanding what is happening in the domain beyond words, the nuances of human interactions. Those who can read the energy of an entire group become empowered as teachers and leaders by knowing just when to push a little further and when to back off to give the group a rest. Spouses sensitive to each other know the optimum times for resolving conflicts and when to leave things alone. They also know each other's subconscious boundaries. Thus, it seems that all human relationships are enhanced by awareness of one's own energy field as well as the field of another person.

Family therapists can certainly attest to the fact of an interactive family energy field. Each family unit seems to have its own unique style, values, patterns of thinking, of acting, and excluding. Watching skilled family therapists at work is akin to watching a master conductor with a diversified group of musicians. Virginia Satir, for instance, was very attuned to the family energy field although she never developed the concept as a definitive theory. In live demonstrations (Evolution of Psychotherapy Conference, Phoenix, AZ, December, 1986) she was constantly smoothing the ruffled feathers of a family member who had been offended or a child that needed to come to focus. She used her hands actively to anchor in the positive qualities of each individual and to disperse the material that was inappropriate. She consciously made herself the ally of the good intent of the family through direct touch and her imposing, energetic presence.

INTERACTIVE BONDING

In healthy relationships, the energy field of one person reaches out and is matched with an equal reaching out from the other. This is the quality of synergy that we discussed earlier in Chapter 4. In therapeutic relationships, the more expanded and focused field of the helper lifts the depleted field of the client to a higher resonance of frequency. In balanced friendships, each person takes turns in alternately being the sender or the receiver of energy. Thus, in a more traditional marriage, the wife sometimes is the caregiver at the end of the week for her exhausted husband; conversely, he takes over when the children become difficult on the weekend. At times the father nurtures and feeds the family, at other times the wife is the primary caregiver. The more flexible these role exchanges are, the healthier and more resilient the relationship will be overall.

Being in love is a unique stage of energy field interaction in which each chakra can be observed to have energetic bands or cords stretching to match the other person's energetic emissions. It is as if very strong energy projections reach out like streamers. Observing people in love is interesting because the energy bonds are so strong they are palpable, even if the couple have not publicly acknowledged their connection.

Sexual union in its highest form arises from the interconnection of all chakras with each other and has a significant impact on the entire field. There is no such thing as "simple sex" or a "one night stand" from an energetic perspective. Beyond physical orgasm, there is emotional interdependence as the fields merge, a fusing of mental patterns, and opportunity for spiritual evolution. The couple literally lift to a higher plane through their interaction, a shared sense of purpose and meaning beyond their ego selves. At its best, this kind of sexual interconnection becomes the generative dynamic for creativity that extends beyond anything the individuals could accomplish by themselves. In a skewed, unequal relationship, unfortunately, this powerful interconnection of energies can lead to dependency, overcompliance, excessive dominance or submission, abuse, and other distortions.

As a healthy relationship matures beyond the initial flush of the interconnecting of all the chakras, the energy fields of the two persons become more separate and full. The bonds continue to exist but there is more flexibility about which ones are activated at a given time. In a mature couple, many things are understood without speaking; they enjoy the depths of their bond and the numerous ways it can be expressed nonverbally.

The parent/child bond is another powerful energy exchange, this time one that evolves and changes considerably over time. Initially, the child is totally dependent, requiring all sustenance from at least one caring adult. Most babies, though, know how to extend their energy fields with smiles and charm to make sure someone responds. The turmoil of adolescence can be seen energetically as one in which the young person's field emerges into its own power and tests the boundaries of the parent's field. If this task is completed successfully, the bond continues throughout adult life as a deep friendship rooted in a history of change. In fact, successful family life seems to be one of the best buffers against the onslaught of change that is so pervasive in our time. Change, within the supportive framework of caring families, can be creative and life-enriching.

The family network of feelings and dreams creates an energetic bond, what we might now call a *family field*. Philosopher and therapist Eric Taub-Bynum writes: "The crucible of our individual psyche is inexorably implicated with each other's psyche. Those we 'know' and resonate with more intensely by intimate and family association spread a matrix that exists within and between us, interlacing us all in an enfolding field . . ." (Taub-Bynum, 1984, p. 203). The pervasive impact of family members on each other has been described by many authors (Wachtel and Wachtel, 1986) and undergirds the application of systems theory to family psychodynamics (Sieberg, 1985). Thus, we view healthy family life as an open system that allows influx of new information and responsiveness to a changing world. In contrast, a closed system, characteristic of an impaired family field, is like a stagnant bay without inflow of new life-waters. In these circumstances we might note enmeshment, poor understanding of boundaries, distortions of bonding, and limited responsiveness to the environment.

DISTORTIONS OF BONDING

As we know too well, there are many possible distortions when human energy fields interact. If one field overpowers the other without awareness or clear intent to help, the result is dominance, manipulation, and control. "Constant vigilance is the price of democracy," observed the French sociologist de Toqueville over 150 years ago. This is also a correct statement of what is needed to maintain energy field balance in relatedness. Each person must be constantly aware not only of her own field and its integrity, but also of what is happening with others' fields.

Our lives are usually filled with dichotomies: male/female, doctor/patient, therapist/client, leader/community, elder/youth, management/labor, privileged/unprivileged, master/slave, and rich/poor, to name only a few. Inequality happens. The resultant dualities and pressures are frequently the norm, the accepted social way of life. It is no wonder, then, that family life, especially the major marital bond, is so filled with inherent pressures.

We are all too familiar with the emotional cost of being enmeshed in someone else's dynamics. Energetically, intuitive persons can actually see these as entangling snares that reach out from the controlling person's field to the unassuming field of another. Barbara Brennan describes them as "bioplasmic streamers" that function like energetic "hooks" (Brennan, 1993, p. 179).

In extreme cases of co-dependency these "hooks" are exceedingly strong, and feel like metal bands on assessment. The constricting bands can impact all the chakras and layers of the energy field. The co-dependent individual literally cannot think for himself. Learning new ways of thinking, feeling, and being can be assisted by therapeutic intervention to help release the "hooks," or overattachments. In the example of Nancy's story in the previous chapter, the entanglement with the father was a pervasive factor in her life. When Nancy began to emerge as a person in her own right, she gradually relinquished the energetic bands, layer by layer, with the assistance of her therapist.

Another form of distortion of human relationship is evidenced energetically by a field that automatically shuts down in certain environments. It is as if the field learns to respond to difficult situations by withdrawing. For some, this may be evidenced by feeling weak in facing the work environment, in hospital settings, or in dealing with large bureaucracies. Initially, it is helpful to recognize and honor the dynamic as a protective reaction. The person may then choose the situations in which she wants to be more effective.

The energetic antidote to withdrawal is expansion and empowerment of the field. In the past, many therapies addressed shyness and introversion with techniques of assertiveness training, role-playing, and anchoring-in of positive feeling states. Energetic maneuvers, such as centering, spinning, and the self-care ideas presented in the next chapter, offer other valuable adjuncts for enhancing the field in difficult settings.

RELATIONSHIP COUNSELING WITH ENERGETIC FOCUS

The energetic focus gives us a new dimension for working with relationship issues. In addition to good cognitive awareness of their dynamics, people in relationships need to find ways of connecting nonverbally. For couples, learning to sense each other's energy and to respond appropriately is invaluable. Bonding even before birth between parents and child is facilitated when the parents learn to sense the baby's energy field and unruffle the area over the mother's abdomen (Krieger, 1993, p. 139) Parent and child relationships can be enhanced by helping the child with day-to-day events such as insomnia or school anxiety.

In very conflicted relationships, the energy bonding offers a way of reaching beyond usual therapy resources. It is as if the energy work allows partners to extend beyond their personalities to lift to a higher Source for solutions.

Betty and John's Story

Betty had suffered from severe depressive disorder for over seven years since college. After a few years of marriage, John, her husband, became so dissatisfied with the relationship that he sought marriage counseling. Betty had been on many different anti-depressants; each would initially provide good results and then diminish in effectiveness as tolerance set in. The couple approached energy healing as a joint venture from which both could learn, even if Betty's condition did not improve. They made a commitment with the therapist to learn as much as they could from each other before considering separation.

Betty and John became intrigued with the possibility of self-care in relation to the human energy field. They started guiding each other through specific practices that helped to enhance the energy field, such as centering and connecting the chakras described in Chapter 10. Progress in Betty's symptom relief was slow but steady. She commented "I still get down, but not as far down as I used to. For someone who has been down a lot, that's an important difference." John benefited as well, noting that he no longer felt entrapped when Betty had one of her "spells." Instead, he could actively work to hold onto his own energetic boundaries during those difficult times.

Currently, Betty and her husband visit their therapist for monthly "maintenance" sessions. They genuinely allow themselves to learn from each other through the bonding that is inherent in their energetic exchanges.

Rita and Marie's Story

Rita and Marie did not come for counseling together; they had not spoken to each other for over eight years. Rita, the mother, had a convoluted life with several marriages, many moves, and constant career changes. When Marie became a teenager, she broke into open rebellion against her mother, called her "stupid," and ran away from home. Many times Rita helped her daughter out of financial difficulties, but the bond between them continued to deteriorate. After Marie married, she broke off all relationship and sent her mother a post card which stated "I am dead to you; do not ever contact me again." Rita carried the emotional burden of the estrangement silently until she heard that Marie had a baby. The flow of tears seemed overwhelming, and it was at that point that Rita sought help. Her field was depleted. There were tight, constrictive bands across the mid-chest and lower pelvis. After allowing her to release her grief, the therapist suggested that Rita send her daughter energetic good wishes from the heart center. Rita later combined her daily heart-centered projections with an image of pink light to surround Marie. She recognized that no power on earth could sever her love for her daughter.

Therapy continued with clearing of the sacral chakra and releasing of the tightly-held bands. Rita expressed the anger and helplessness of her situation. Beyond that, however, she started to recognize she still had choices to make within herself. She could feel victimized by Marie's hardness, or she could express who she was, including her caring for Marie and the grandchild.

The heart center opened more and more while Rita externalized the image of her daughter. In her therapy, she told Marie what she thought, and sent Marie to her own light to get whatever she needed to heal. Eventually, Rita decided to send a simple written note to Marie about the baby, being careful not to have any expectations or attachments to the outcome.

A month later, Marie called her mother, saying, "I don't know what's happening, but you've been on my mind a lot. Thank you for your card and good wishes." The relationship is still strained; it may take years to resolve, or it may never progress, but somehow an opening has been made. A small light now shines in the darkness.

INTENTIONALITY AND INTUITION

Any time a person works with another's energy field there is a subtle but noticeable effect. For this reason centering, clearly setting one's intent to help another, is the most essential step in any interactive work. When the healer enters the energy field of a client, the full intent to help by focusing on the client is essential. Similarly, when the healer withdraws her hands from the field, the intent needs to be for closure. The purpose is to complete the interaction at that time. If this is not done, the recipient of the intervention may feel abandoned or otherwise disconnected from the healer. Most of the time, interaction from helper to recipient is characterized by the helper's hands being in the "allow mode," that is, sensing and following the energy. The process of following the client's energy flow using the sense of touch allows a hot area of the field to cool, a congested area to flow, a cold area to warm up, or a bumpy, irregular portion of the field to become smoother.

Clear agreement about energetic signals becomes the foundation of a trust that can develop between energy healer and client, between parent and child, and between committed partners. If the person receiving an energetic intervention is unable to respond verbally or nonverbally, as in the case of an infant or someone who is dying, then the healer needs to deeply attune to her own intuition. In these instances, she must exhibit a willingness to do what seems helpful under guidance from her own inner healer, paying close attention to the client's response, and repeating the intervention as necessary when it is evaluated to be effective.

ASSISTING WITH BIRTHING AND DYING

Another powerful opportunity for utilizing energy field ideas exists in supporting families who are undergoing major life transitions, including the process of giving birth or surrendering a family member to death. During these times, the healer can assist with the freeing, or expansion of the field. This would be true for the days or hours preceding death as well as during the months of preparation for the birth of a new member. In either of these situations, the therapist can support the flow of energy which moves wherever it is most needed. Of prime importance during these sacred moments is the intention of the caregiver. Being deeply centered allows the healer to hold a peaceful focus during times of major family changes.

Chris' Story: A Time for Birth

One of our colleagues lived in a remote mountain area where she befriended a lovely country woman named Chris, her husband, and 9-year-old son. They were a self-sufficient family with a love for the simple aspects of life and a firm religious foundation. Chris was pregnant with her second child and prepared for the long-awaited dream of giving birth at home. Chris engaged a local midwife and sought out the therapist to meet with the family for several pre-birth counseling sessions.

When Chris approached her due date, she did not appear ready to give birth. Two weeks passed without any change. The therapist was asked to assist with energy healing. She found the field open in relation to the upper part of the body, but closed in the lower part, as if Chris was literally holding the baby in. The therapist cleared the field until it became smooth and symmetrical and suggested that Chris call if anything further was needed.

The following week there was still no baby, but instead a very agitated Chris. The physician in attendance had apparently suggested hospitalizing Chris to monitor the fetus and to ensure that nothing was wrong. Chris was distressed about the physician's seemingly heavy-handed approach. She sensed that the baby was fine, but her concerns and fears were increasing.

When the therapist came at the couple's request, she placed her hands over Chris' belly, smoothing the area repeatedly. As she did this, the energy field visibly expanded. Karilee encouraged Chris to smooth her own field and to talk to the baby directly. While doing this, Chris burst into tears. "I'm sorry, I'm so sorry," she repeated several times while sobbing and holding her large abdomen. Husband and son entered the room alarmed at the crying, which was very rare in their household. The therapist encouraged them to gently add their hands to the smoothing of the mother and baby's energy fields. Chris heaved a sigh and continued to express her grief.

Chris told the baby that she was afraid, something she had been reluctant to admit even to herself. She explained between sobs that the last birth had been so difficult that she was afraid to go through a similar experience. Her husband stroked her head gently, bringing her back to full awareness. She looked into the eyes of her dear son who held her while she talked about his difficult birth. She smiled with pure love at them both, and laughter began to mingle with the tears. Clearly, there was now an energetic bond between all of them. Soon the whole room was alive with vibrant energy.

Suddenly, Chris' face registered a change. Imagine the surprise of all around when Chris went into labor spontaneously!

The midwife was called, and the little girl was born within two hours. No one was more surprised, however, than the doctor. The following day Chris walked into his office at the time of her appointment with a baby girl in her arms.

Several weeks later, Chris described how her fear seemed to bind the energy flow in the abdomen and birth canal. The energetic intervention helped to loosen the hold of the embedded fear from the past. This process of releasing, coupled with verbal expression of the fear, provided a catalyst for a gentle and uneventful birth. It is not likely that energetic maneuvers by themselves would have caused the baby to arrive earlier, but rather that Chris was finally ready to release her blocked pattern and to move forward with the powerful life experience of giving birth.

Rod's Story: A Time to Die

Rod was in his late thirties when he was diagnosed a second time with cancer. After his first bout with throat cancer years earlier, he had been declared cancer-free, and fathered two children with his wife Lora. Both became extremely stressed with parenting responsibilities, turbulent marital discord, financial difficulty, and the death of their 5-month-old child due to a birth defect. This time, Rod sought out a therapist to support him in battling his disease.

Work with his multidimensional energy field was incorporated throughout the counseling relationship. First, he addressed inner conflicts related to his difficult childhood and lack of intimacy through the energetic release sequence (described in Chapter 7). Then, he began to consolidate his relationship with his wife. Lora began attending the sessions and learned how to assist in clearing his energy field, especially after chemotherapy. A deep bond grew between them as a result. Together they developed a video and notebook for couples to use in dealing with cancer. Soon it became apparent that Rod was not going to improve. The energy work helped both of them to access the transpersonal domain more fully and to prepare for a meaningful, conscious transition.

When the time came for Rod to pass on, he was surrounded by his loving wife, his child, and many friends. He was well-respected for his courage, both for the passion with which he had lived his life, and for being able to surrender to death. He had grown immeasurably as a person and felt spiritually connected to his greater purpose. Rod and Lora worked out methods of communicating beyond physical death, giving them both a sense of mastery surrounding this final evolution of the soul. Rather than being fearful, they were curious, eager to learn, and centered as they faced the mystery of his dying. No longer fighting, Rod released his body gently, as his wife cleared the area from the center of each chakra outward to help expand his energy field. She felt him lift and let go, and finally, with a deep sigh, move beyond physical life. Those gathered around were deeply touched. All of them participated in focusing their hands, hearts, and breath to facilitate Rod's final healing.

After Rod left his body, an energy healer guided those present to breathe fully and deeply, to balance their own fields. The fear that often surrounds death in our culture was transformed: each person was touched by the energy of this powerful event. Rod's child kissed him on the forehead, announcing that Dad was with the little brother. Tears of sadness mixed with songs as music filled the room in accordance with Rod's wishes that a celebration be held. His energy.continued to assist his friends long after his departure.

SUMMARY

In this chapter we have looked at human relationships from an energetic perspective. The ability to understand the impact of field interaction can be a valuable adjunct to family and relationship counseling. In addition, energy work has much to offer in assisting with complex family conflicts, increasing sensitivity, and awareness. Energy balancing is sometimes the only way of reaching out to a loved one in times of physical separation or in the complex transitions of birthing and dying.

REFERENCES

Brennan, B. *Light Emerging*. (1993) New York: Bantam Books.

Krieger, D. *Accepting Your Power to Heal*. Santa Fe, NM: Bear and Co., p. 138–143, 1993.

Wachtel, E., and Wachtel, P. *Family Dynamics in Individual Psychotherapy: A Guide to Clinical Strategies*. New York: Guildford Press, p. 43–64 1986.

Sieberg, E. *Family Communications: An Integrated Systems Approach*. New York: Gardner Press, p. 32–55 1985.

Taub-Bynum, E. B. *The Family Unconscious*. Wheaton, IL: Quest Books, 1984.

V | DEVELOPMENT OF THE HEALER

In this section we address an issue that is seldom considered in the therapeutic literature: the personal care and development of the helper. Whether the reader is a consumer or a health care professional, the principles of self-care and their application in practice require full attention and commitment.

In Chapter 14 specific ideas and exercises for care of the personal energy field are brought forth. In Chapter 15 we look at the therapist's ethics of caregiving, especially when using energy healing concepts. Chapter 16 sums up the many intriguing worlds of psychoenergy healing in therapy that we have explored, with an invitation to further extend our vision into the future.

14

CARE OF THE HEALER: MAINTAINING BALANCE IN ONE'S OWN FIELD

All healing, whether in the physical or emotional realm, is self-healing: actual change always comes from within. The spark of insight that changes an attitude, a thinking pattern, or neuropeptides in the complex functions of the physical body must be ignited within each of us if healing is to occur. The work of the caregiver, whether nurse, physician, therapist, educator, or loved one, is to activate the client's self-healing capacity. In order to do this, we ourselves are in need of balancing and healing.

One person who addressed the inherent principle of self-healing was Florence Nightingale, the mid-nineteenth century spiritual philosopher, statistician, and founder of modern nursing. "Nature alone cures," she wrote, "and what nursing has to do . . . is to put the patient in the best condition for nature to act upon him." (Nightingale, 1969, p. 133). Her insistence upon opening up the confined, dark hospitals of her day to plenty of sunlight, flow of fresh air, nutrition, fluid balance, spiritual expression, and emotional support predates our current holistic paradigm by a century and a half. She was a pioneer in asserting the right of each person to adequate care and self-determination, whether he was a patient or a caregiver (Calabria and Macrae, 1994).

Further, Jung felt that if people did not deal with the powerful forces within, they would live with a potentially destructive shadow that could overpower the waking consciousness. If we are to be truly effective facilitators of someone's healing journey, we must be willing to experience our own inner turmoil and its resolution in all aspects of our lives. Only through our own processes do we become competent to assist others in their struggles. The psychotherapist becomes the "shaman," the bearer of the healing archetype, who walks between the worlds, supporting individuals as they rummage through the collective human psyche and interpret the meaning of symbols on their own personal odyssey. "The person who commits himself to a life of continuing confrontation with the unconscious within himself, will also confront the unknown in the world at large with an open mind, and what is more, with a heart of wisdom" (Jung, 1964, p. 227). These words remind us of our commitment, as client and therapist, in our search for meaning and healing.

In the current era of consumer-directed care, we recognize the vast potential each of us has for self-healing when there is appropriate external support. For example, all of us have ongoing inner dialogue that can be helpful in facing issues and exploring options. The familiar cliche was "If you talk to yourself, you need help." More recent psychological thinking actually holds that the lack of inner dialogue, and its accompanying inner processing, leads to emotional problems. Thus, it is more accurate to say "If you don't talk to yourself in a productive, caring way, you need help." The important thing is the nature of the inner dialogue. Is it creative and nurturing? Or is it critical, judging, ruminating, or shaming?

We notice that our conscious awareness has different parts, akin to the three major ego states identified by Eric Berne, founder of Transactional Analysis (Berne, 1975). He labeled these aspects of ourselves the Critical and Nurturing Parent, the Adult, or the Adaptive and Natural Child. Another approach is to simply call the parts by their functions. Thus, parent and child dialogue can be internal, within ourselves, as well as descriptive of an external, current relationship. Similarly, there can be internal discussion between our own fearful and comforting personalities, and our basic needs and the Higher Self, our inner client and therapist.

The reconciliation of these internal parts is the task of the inner healer. Self-care requires listening to the disputing voices within and moving to a higher perspective for resolution. One way of activating our inner healing voice is to connect with a sense of the inner advisor or personal guidance (discussed in Chapter 8 on imagery). Another is to pay attention to early signs of energetic depletion and then use our hands and heart, through centering and alignment with the infinite resources of the Universal Energy Field, to help bring about more balance. We will explore some specific ways to accomplish this as we proceed.

BURNOUT FROM AN ENERGETIC PERSPECTIVE

Burnout describes a condition of being so overwhelmed by the needs of others that the caregiver himself can no longer cope adequately. Thinking becomes stultified, and even simple tasks take longer and longer to perform. In short, the caregiver becomes ineffective in helping others. The phenomenon of burnout has been studied and described in the social sciences literature, as in nurse Snow's aptly titled book *I'm Dying to Take Care of You* (Snow and Willard, 1989) and Schaef's *The Addictive Organization* (Schaef and Fassel, 1988). In energetic terms, we would say that burnout results when the individual energy centers, and finally the entire field of the caregiver become depleted.

The field is our tool for facilitating the flow of energy on behalf of our clients and ourselves. Maintaining field integrity and balance is primary. Our emotions, and their related energy layers, are like antennae, sensors that give us feedback when something is amiss. As we learn to trust the emotions and the intuition associated with them we have rapid moment-by-moment feedback about ourselves, others, and our environment. Awareness, coupled with kindly inner dialogue, is often sufficient to resolve a dilemma.

We now have the additional resource of paying attention to each of the energy centers. Most of us have one or several centers that are especially vulnerable in stressful situations. For example, Alice became afraid, passive, and tired every time her boss spoke in a harsh voice. The accompanying depletion of the root chakra meant that she literally had no resources for countering the stimulus. Charging up her sense of vitality with the Energetic Spin (described in Chapter 11) became an effective alternative to helpless passivity. The sense of increasing energy, coupled with affirmations and assertiveness skills, empowered Alice to practice looking directly at her boss, stating how she felt, and giving more empowered responses.

Each chakra emits signals that can be felt early, at the beginning of energetic depletion. The heart center, for example, begins to close when we feel tightness in the chest or are unable to take a full, deep breath. The earliest sign of throat chakra depletion is a frog in the throat or a change in the tone of voice while speaking. These signals give us an opportunity to modulate energy over the depleted center or to spin through the entire field. By paying attention to the first twinge of an incipient headache with clearing movements, we can help the affected area become more balanced before a full headache develops. Since physical symptoms most often follow emotional distress and its accompanying energetic depletion, we are provided with excellent tools in energy awareness for preventing illness in its earliest stages.

SELF-CARE THROUGH THE HUMAN ENERGY FIELD

Energy field self-care requires beginning the intervention at the very first signal and repeating it as often as needed. As self-knowledge increases, you may find that only a hint of tiredness or shallow breathing quickly leads you to institute energetic maneuvers. Thus, *awareness* of the drop in our energy level is the first step. *Centering* immediately when we sense energetic depletion follows. Then, we can actively work to *release* the tension from the field and to set our conscious intent to *align* with our higher purpose and goals. We *notice* at the same time any aspect of our personal agendas, conscious or subconscious, that may be depleting or limiting this alignment. With such careful *self-monitoring* we can feel better and better, more alive, and creative. Several exercises are listed below for self-care, in addition to the ones we have already suggested, for maintaining your vital energy field.

Exercise: Centering Through the Heart

Since the heart energy center establishes our connection with others, it is perhaps most challenged by the day-to-day work with emotionally needy persons. Feeling connected heart-to-heart with another person, without demands or expectations, is a major challenge for health care professionals.

1. Begin by visualizing the most beautiful emerald green you have ever seen. Let your mind's eye travel into deep northern forests, to tropical jungles, to lush new plants by a soothing stream, or visualize an emerald crystal.

2. Allow this color to bathe your heart, the mid-chest area, and lungs with a comforting and nurturing feeling. Sense the support of the beauty of nature for your being. Breathe fully and deeply, releasing any darkness or constrictions with the out-breath.

3. Allow yourself to see someone who loves you deeply in front of you. Feel the vibration of that person's caring. Now let the love-light from your heart center reach out to the person, letting go of any resentments that might still be lingering in the relationship. Experience the rich fullness of your shared energy fields.

4. Feeling nourished and supported, begin to see your own being, perhaps earlier, at a trying time in your life. Allow the same intensity of love and forgiveness to flow to this younger self, comforting and acknowledging the lessons you are learning from the difficult past experience.

5. Hold the heart area with your hands while continuing to feel the flow of caring for yourself in this area.

6. If other energy centers feel depleted, let the same warming touch go to each of them.

7. Feel your entire energy field smooth and balance; state your goals for the day and move forward, continuing to feel the warmth in your heart area.

Exercise: Chakra Meditation

As we discussed in Chapter 5, each chakra has a psychological meaning. Awareness of the energy centers that are most vulnerable, or easily closed, gives us a tremendous tool for self-enhancement. The following exercise has as many creative variations as you wish to use, including your own imagery and affirmations.

1. See the color of each energy center, starting with red at the root and moving through to the green of the heart center and the subtle expanding purple, violet, orchid, silver, and gold of the crown and transpersonal centers. See the whole rainbow of your energies in all its radiance and splendor.

2. Modulate energy over the lower three centers while working, one at a time, with an affirmation related to the Will to Live, the Will to Feel, and the Will to Think. See the lower three chakras as a triangle of light supporting you, grounding you so that you can move to the upper levels with ease.

3. Modulate energy over the heart center, the transformational center of the Will to Love with unconditional acceptance and caring. Note how this center is supported by the lower triangle so that your awareness can move higher to accomplish its task.

4. Modulate energy over the upper three centers, affirming in turn the Will to Self-Expression, the Will to Intuition, and the Will to Fulfillment aligned with your highest purpose. See the upper three centers as an inverted triangle that expands beyond your personal being to the transpersonal dimension.

5. Sense your whole being as connected through an inner core of golden light that touches each of the chakras and the Universal Energy Field. Allow yourself to feel firm and steadfast while moving on with grace and flexibility to your next task or endeavor.

6. Thank yourself for taking this time to reconfirm and declare your inner direction.

Exercise: Release Rituals

Often, a simple brushing down with the hands over the shoulders, the back, the front, and the legs is all that is needed to disconnect from a difficult situation. Shaking out arms, hands, legs, and feet can be done in addition. If you sense a strong emotion while doing this, you may want to add an image, such as a baseball flying past outfield, to assist with letting go. If the strong emotion lingers, you are receiving feedback that there is further work to be done, either through your journal-izing or with help from a trusted person, to process and re-lease the disturbance.

Practice designing your own rituals to release the ten-sions of your work. Use this ritual before, during, and after every workday or challenging encounter.

Do something for each of the four major layers of the en-ergy field.

1. For the physical body, relax muscle groups.

2. For the emotional body, discharge, blow out, and let go.

3. For the mental body, bring in a healing thought or image.

4. For the spiritual body, connect with your inner peace through silence and by visualizing the inner core of your light aligned with the Infinite.

Exercise: Connecting to the Transpersonal Perspective

One of the strongest benefits of energy-oriented interventions is the direct connection of our finite energies with the infinite supply of energy surrounding us, as exemplified in nature. When we align with the Universal Energy Field we tap into our higher awareness, expanding our options to unlimited po-tential. The following exercise is a sample of the myriad ways you could enhance your transpersonal perspective in addition to the suggestions offered in Chapter 9.

1. Allow yourself to be relaxed and comfortable with pen and paper at your side. Take a few breaths and let any heaviness release fully.

2. Connect with a perceived conflict, whether at work, in your family, or possibly even one experienced in a dream. Write down the position you identify as your own at the bottom corner of a triangle. Describe the feelings associated with your point of view.

3. Write down the position of the other person at the other bottom corner of the triangle. Imagine fully what it would be like to be in the other person's shoes for

the moment. Write all the feelings you could imagine for the other person.

4. Note how each party is correct in some way. Step back from the material level of the conflict and allow your awareness to shift to the apex of the triangle. What larger framework could encompass the possibility of both parties being right?

5. Imagine yourself as one of your most honored teachers. Move as high as possible. What would this teacher say? How could each party be honored and come to a negotiated peace? Allow your inner advisor to assist you in writing down at least three available solutions.

6. After writing, sense the expansion of your energy field to include your connection to Higher Power and Infinite Potential. Ask if the three possible solutions mesh with your highest ideal. If so, proceed with practical ways of putting the ideas into action. If not, go back to your inner guidance for more options at the apex of the triangle and repeat the process.

7. Thank your inner being for willingness to explore new options through alignment with the Higher Self. Let yourself repeat the process daily until this problem and others come to resolution.

LIMITATIONS OF SELF-CARE

Since centering is the focal point of energetic self-care, inability to hold a centered state of awareness would be a major limitation. Severe physical pain can cloud all dimensions of the field in such a way that clear thinking, let alone focusing, are impossible. Emotional pressures can also be so distracting that one is literally "caught up" in the compelling feelings, unable to see clearly. We also recognize the power of our own denial and projections that can literally blind us to aspects of ourselves that may be very obvious to someone else. It makes sense, then, to seek appropriate helpers whenever we are in such states to assist with the balancing of our energies. The assistance might well include medication for pain relief or expressive release work.

Fortunately, there are increasing numbers of creative medical, body-oriented, and psychological professionals to help when our self-care capacity is diminished. If these helpers are genuine, they will facilitate access to our own healing resources as soon as the crisis has been resolved.

PERSONAL DEVELOPMENT SUGGESTIONS

There are easily thousands of ways that each caregiver can develop more personal awareness. We have suggested working with your own internal imagery related to the chakras and meditations that include the various layers of the energy field. Specific disciplines, including Yoga, Chi Qung, Tai Chi, and dance (Dossey et al., 1988) are especially effective because they activate the entire energy field, allowing thought to focus through repetitive movement. In addition, writing a journal is a practical way of bringing thoughts into action. Creative self-expression through play, music, drawing mandalas, or working with clay and plants (Hover-Kramer et al., 1996), can be powerful tools for self-discovery to appreciate the depth of your being in all dimensions.

Whatever you choose, let it become a part of your daily practice. There should be some activity in each day that gives joy and satisfaction. In addition, there should be some daily way of taking inventory of the personal energy field to bring in selected interventions for restoring balance and wholeness.

SUMMARY

Our goal as therapists is for effective self-healing so we can be transparent facilitators of energy flow for our clients. We move from recognition of personal emotional issues, and temporary dependence on others, to effective self-care. This is especially evident when we work with our own energy fields. Because of the rapid self-awareness that develops, we can release emotional constrictions from the field and move to higher levels of functioning.

REFERENCES

Berne, E. *Transactional Analysis in Psychotherapy*. New York: Grove Press, 1961.

Calabria, M., and Macrae, J. (eds.). *Suggestions for Thought by Florence Nightingale.* Philadelphia, PA: University of Pennsylvania Press, 1994.

Dossey, B. et al. *Holistic Nursing Handbook.* Rockville, MD: Aspen Publishers, 1988, p. 169–170.

Hover-Kramer, D. et al. *Healing Touch.* Albany, NY: Delmar Publishers, 1996, p. 213–225.

Nightingale, F. *Notes on Nursing.* London: Harrison, 1859. Reprint. New York: Dover, 1969.

Schaef, A.W., and Fassel, D. *The Addictive Organization.* San Francisco: Harper and Row, 1988.

Snow, C., and Willard, D. *I'm Dying to Take Care of You.* Redmond, WA: Professional Counselor Books, 1989.

ETHICAL CONSIDERATIONS FOR ENERGY HEALING

An ethic of care involves a morality grounded in relationship and response.

—Rita Manning (1992)

Ethics is a set of values, a code for translating the moral into daily life."

—Rachel Naomi Remen (1988)

Beyond written rules and the law, ethical principles guide therapeutic interaction to bring forth positive, life-enhancing outcomes. The healing relationship is a unique interchange in which the therapist's values become translated into her presence and responsiveness. The therapist's internal congruence is grounded in her sense of integrity and her knowledge base. The therapist's external congruence is made visible by consciously choosing a definable code of ethics and values. As each discipline in the social sciences has developed, so has its corresponding code of ethics in the fields of psychology (1992), feminist therapy (1991), music therapy (1994), holotropic breathwork (1994), and marriage and family counseling (1991).

Whenever there is a major shift in thinking, as we are seeing with the holistic framework and complementary modalities such as energy healing, a new code of ethics must also emerge. The rapidly developing field of holistic health care, and the expanded definitions of healing suggested in Chapter 1 require ethical considerations that invite us to stretch our thinking and expand our awareness. So far in this volume we have viewed concepts related to the practice of energy healing. As we consider ethics and standards of care, we see the work coming to life in its unique form, as a major contribution to the health care field.

Kylea Taylor, a Holotropic Breathwork facilitator, authored a significant new book, entitled the *Ethics of Caring: Honoring the Web of Life in Our Professional Healing Relationships* (1995). This book addresses ethical considerations related to the many emerging complementary therapies. These new therapies include work with nonordinary states of consciousness such as guided imagery, hypnotherapy, art therapy, dreamwork, age regression, and others. Although energy healing is not mentioned specifically, it is likewise an emerging modality in which nonordinary states of consciousness appear spontaneously, requiring specific skills on the part of the caregiver.

Taylor's definition of ethics is closely aligned with the holistic model we have discussed: "Ethical behavior is reverence for life demonstrated by right relationship to another" (Taylor, 1995, p. 10). Right relationship in energy healing means bringing the awareness of subtle energies into all aspects of the therapeutic exchange. Beyond the usual client/therapist agreements—i.e., mutual goal setting, confidentiality, truth-telling, injunctions against any sexual expression, nonharming, agreements about fees, meetings, and time and place—much more is required to promote an ethical practice of energy healing. In addition to all the usual concerns listed, there must be sensitivity about appropriate use of intuitive material. The helper may find herself connecting clairvoyantly with the client's energy field, even to the extent of sensing the client's pain which can create additional hazards of countertransference. On the other hand, the client may project his spiritual ideals onto the therapist, creating increased possibility of transference and unrealistic expectations. Thus, careful attention to boundaries is even more crucial in energy-related counseling than in talk therapies. In fact, total respect for the client's process and pace is a requirement for those using this noninvasive modality.

WORKING WITH NONORDINARY STATES OF CONSCIOUSNESS

States of consciousness that move us to deeper levels of inner awareness beyond ordinary consensus reality can be accessed in a variety of ways. Within the context of energy healing, the simple shift to deeper relaxation in a safe environment may be enough to help the client experience internal images or to connect with a repressed memory. This change in perception can allow intense experiences to arise that are known by various names in the psychotherapy literature: therapeutic breakthroughs, altered states, peak experiences, abreaction, catharsis, or regression. The term, *nonordinary state of consciousness* is used by Taylor to describe these phenomena "because it is a broad, nonjudgmental term which includes any state of consciousness characterized by heightened sensitivity" (1995, p. 13). She describes ordinary awareness with eyes open, usual perception of time, self, and others, and differentiates it from mild and deeper states of nonordinary consciousness in which reverie increases and reference points to everyday reality such as time, place, and verbal expression decrease markedly.

As suggested in the chapter on transpersonal perspectives, nonordinary states have great therapeutic potential because they allow the client to transcend his limited self-concept with redefinition of himself and expansion of boundaries. At the same time, the client is in a state of enhanced suggestibility, allowing for any gesture or voice inflection from the therapist to be internalized without his usual defenses. It is as if the healer's energy field becomes visible to the client who is in a state of heightened sensitivity. The client may even sense the thought form in the helper's aura as described by clairvoyants (Leadbeater, 1980; Brennan, 1987). If there is any hint of nonacceptance regarding the client's emotionally charged issues such as abuse, birth memories, or past life experiences, the client may halt his inner process or internalize the perceived criticism. Thus, the healer's intent, motivation, and self-understanding become part of the client's experience. Any limitation in the helper's energies communicates directly with the client's field.

Suggestions of Abuse

As the client accesses nonverbal imagery, repressed memories often surface. Within the realities of therapeutic uncertainty, these memories may be historically true, partially true, or constructed to compensate for gaps in personal history. The sense of having been abused may also be symbolic in nature. This confusing combination of materials reported by the client requires exquisite caution on the part of the therapist. Allowing the client to release intrapsychic pressure associated with submerged issues by energetic clearing is helpful and necessary. Action based on internal material as if it were totally factual is not always desirable, nor is it helpful (Ross, 1995).

A neutral, noninvasive approach is especially valuable in light of recent debates on "false memory syndrome." Many therapists have fallen into the trap of suggesting possibilities of sexual abuse to the client who cannot remember his childhood (Yapko, 1994). Because the human brain functions similar to a hologram, clients may take such suggestions and construct a memory to fill in missing details. Unfortunately, this opens the door to wild conjecture and accusations concerning events that may not have actually happened in the individual's personal history. Abuse and victimization are definitely historical realities that form part of our collective memory as human beings.

The American Psychiatric Association's ethics statement on memories of sexual abuse (1994) offers an appropriate response for therapists:

> It is not known how to distinguish, with complete accuracy, memories based on true events from those derived from other sources. . . . Some patients will be left with unclear memories of abuse and no corroborating information . . . treatment may help these patients adapt to the uncertainty regarding such emotionally important issues.

Integration and Closure

Another ethical concern in working with nonordinary states of consciousness involves the therapist's intentional effort to assist the client with integration and closure of his experiences. Completion after any session of energy healing is crucial. Assimilation of the inner experience can be facilitated by taking at least the last third of a therapy session for discussion and making sure the client has returned to ordinary car-driving alertness. Holding the hands or feet at the close of a session, or encouraging the client to dance and move about, further facilitates the client's grounding to the earth and consensus reality. Space-time orientation can be facilitated by having the client pay specific attention to the physical environment, such as counting pictures on the wall or describing furniture details.

The therapist also needs to help bridge the client's conversations about his experience, particularly with others who are not equally attuned to higher sense perception of subtle energies. In many traditions of therapy, having visions and an inner advisor would be considered pathological, especially if the client were to try to make his inner reality concrete in the external world. The caregiver must assist the client to prevent misunderstandings about his inner work and help orient him to effective communication with others. Material from the inner realm is best handled by clients who have the flexibility of thinking that allows them to distinguish when it is appropriate to share personal material from when it is not.

COMPETENCIES REQUIRED FOR ENERGY-RELATED HEALING

Multidimensional healing requires specific competencies, skills, and knowledge in addition to the development of higher sense perception and intuition. Although techniques may be relatively easy to learn, the principles and foundations supporting appropriate applications are more complex. We will discuss the training and supervision involved in the work, the need for clarity about physical touching, and the need to maintain clear boundaries that enhance the facilitator's personal awareness.

Clarity About Physical Touch

All persons who communicate with others need to be clear about physical touch and its appropriate use. Energy healing per se does not require physical touching, since the human energy field extends well beyond the physical body. All approaches suggested in this book can be done by moving the hands above the body in the client's energy field. This fact gives energy healing many advantages beyond physical therapies such as massage or acupuncture. Energy clearing and balancing can be performed in proximity to a physical area that may be too painful to touch or above a part of the body where direct contact would be inappropriate.

Energy healing work is done with the client fully clothed while resting on a comfortable recliner or couch. Some practitioners prefer to use massage tables; it is a matter of personal choice, not a necessity. The therapist is usually seated next to the client so she can reach the client's field easily with her hands. Some therapists have found the use of a blanket helpful. This serves to provide an added sense of protection and comfort as well as to prevent the cooling of the client's body temperature that accompanies deeper states of relaxation.

Because the light, caring touch that can be used in energy healing is often very comforting, many clients ask to be touched, especially when they feel a sense of trust and bonding. The wise counselor clarifies the client's preferences about physical contact at the beginning of the therapeutic relationship. At the same time, the therapist needs to be aware of the ways touch has been misused in the client's past, for punishment or inappropriate sexual contact, and respect the client's preferences. Sometimes, healer intuition is the only guidance available. It is wise to trust one's intuition, or simply said "When in doubt, leave it out." Respect for the integrity of the client's field is first and foremost .

Within the framework of humanistic caring, we recognize that while touch can be misused, there are also many times that it would be inappropriate *not* to touch. For example, a lack of physical touching might further exacerbate the sense of abandonment or rejection experienced in the client's childhood. Many individuals, especially the isolated and elderly, are touch-deprived, starving for a sense of tangible connection with others. Taylor observes (1995, p. 60):

> Ordinary therapy may be very adequate most of the time without the therapist touching the client. There. are times when a therapist should not touch a client; therefore, some have made it unethical ever to touch the client. This logic is flawed. It ignores those times when it is important to touch a client even during ordinary therapy. When we are working with a client in a nonordinary state of consciousness, there are some occasions when *not* touching the client would be unethical.

Training and Supervision

Currently, there are many programs that teach energy healing. These include Therapeutic Touch which is supported by the

Nurse Healers—Professional Associates; Healing Touch, pioneered by the American Holistic Nurses' Association; the Barbara Brennan School of Healing Science; and Rosalyn Bruyere's Crucible Program, to name just a few (for a more complete listing see Appendix A). The psychotherapy track within the Transformational Pathways™ Program of Multidimensional Healing is uniquely designed for practicing psychotherapists and requires licensure in one's state for acceptance.

Most training to provide a safe practice of energy healing occurs over a period of two or more years with repeated opportunities for experiential learning. This requirement of learning energetic interventions through personal experience is comparable to the supervised practices built into counseling education programs, and to the tradition that required anyone seeking to become a psychoanalyst to first be analyzed. Persons wishing to develop healership must have direct knowledge of their own breakthroughs in order to help clients chart the course through the unknown waters of the subconscious psyche. If the healer has no knowledge of this inner territory, she would have no way of helping clients to normalize or integrate their own experiences.

Supervision and regular contact with colleagues is another important aspect of effective healership. Every healer must be willing to explore his own motivation, his distractions, and the many elements of caring through regular consultation. A list of psychotherapists who have advanced experience with energy healing is available through the Holistic Alliance of Professional Practitioners, Entrepreneurs and Networkers, Inc. (HAPPEN), included in Appendix A.

Maintaining Boundaries

As has already been implied, the counselor must maintain a clear sense of boundaries in energy field interactions. "If we have unhealthy boundaries, we can be like sponges that absorb the painful, conflicted material [of the client]" (Whitfield, 1993, p. 248). Because client issues may resonate with similar patterns in the healer's field, knowing one's personal fears and limitations and their relation to each energy center is essential (Taylor, 1995). Otherwise, the helper could misuse the very strengths of the subtle energies to distort desired outcomes.

For example, a helper with unclear boundaries may become enmeshed in the client's third chakra issues. The client may ask for advice and appear helpless in decision-making; the healer, wishing to be resourceful, influences client decisions in covert ways. An insidious pattern is set up in which the healer begins to associate her wish to make a difference in the client's life with her own sense of power and status. Ultimately, this can lead to increased client dependency and a heightened sense of powerlessness.

IMPLICATIONS FOR PRACTICE

There are many implications for practice in the concerns we have brought forth. Some of the most important involve establishing selection criteria for appropriate clients, ensuring informed consent, and defining the scope of one's practice.

Selection of Clients for Energetic Approaches

Some clients are not appropriate for entering work that may involve nonordinary states of consciousness. This includes persons who are generally suspicious, who have thought disorders, who have severe personality dissociation, or who have not developed a sense of trust with their facilitator. Others are individuals who have strong opinions against unconventional therapies. Clients with poor ego boundaries or very fragile self-esteem may likewise be poor candidates because they lack the flexibility to make shifts between ordinary and nonordinary states of consciousness. Similarly, the very stressed, tired, or overwhelmed may simply be too confused by intrapsychic material to benefit from energetic approaches until their lives are more stabilized.

Ideal clients for energy healing are those who have an active interest in extending awareness of their inner lives, and those who express curiosity about this form of therapy. The client needs to be able to tolerate the paradox between his current external life and the images with which he makes contact internally. Without this, the cognitive dissonance may be too great and lead to further distress. As we have illustrated in the case examples, energetic interventions facilitate rapid breakthroughs that may not be achieved as readily with verbal therapy alone. Adequate, nonjudgmental emotional support through these times is essential. At other times, deeper insights may come days or weeks after an energy healing session, and clients must know that contact with the therapist is available to them. It is crucial to respect the clients' pace and to proceed with care, following the client's cues at every step.

Informed Consent

Informed consent means ensuring that each client knows the benefits and risks of the modality that is being used. In relation to energy healing the benefits are many: deep levels of relaxation; a sense of personal empowerment; accessing repressed material; rich therapeutic imagery; communication beyond words; and connecting with the transpersonal perspective, to name a few.

Each of these benefits has some inherent risk. For example, increased self-awareness allows for new ways of looking at patterns in one's life and could result in dissatisfaction with things as they are. It is important, then, to discuss therapeutic goals at the outset and to re-evaluate goals frequently in light of emerging material as the client progresses. The risks of changing one's life can only be correctly assessed by the client himself; the counselor, however, can help to assess readiness and timing.

There are no known instances of therapeutic harm or energy field overdose in relation to the healing concepts outlined in this book. The ethic of caring and rapport between the therapist and client energy fields requires continuous monitoring and attention.

A sample informed consent form used by Energy Healers is illustrated in Appendix C. The items on the form can lead to further discussion when the client is considering this complementary modality.

Defining the Scope of Practice

Another way we can clarify the ideas we have put forth here is to compare energy-oriented interventions and their outcomes with other known approaches to the subconscious mind. It is important for all therapists to define their scope of practice by differentiating clearly what they can offer and what is outside their expertise.

Energy healing seems to access profound synthesis and integration in clients who are comfortable with nonordinary states of consciousness. There are many avenues for reaching nonordinary states of awareness. A comparison with two other methods, meditation and hypnotherapy, allows us another way of appreciating the unique contributions of psychoenergetic healing.

Rather than viewing all states of nonordinary awareness as being the same, we notice marked differences between meditation, energy healing, and hypnotherapy. We might say that meditation and hypnotherapy are at opposite ends of the spectrum because meditation is almost totally self-directed whereas hypnotherapy is clearly initiated and mediated by a highly skilled practitioner. In meditation, there are many different levels of consciousness, ranging from merely quieting mental chatter to advanced stages of insight and peace after years of deepening spiritual practice (Walsh, 1995). In hypnotherapy, a deep altered state of consciousness is induced by the practitioner, and the client is willing, in effect, to be temporarily dependent on the therapist for therapeutic outcomes.

In a practice of energy-related healing, the client's experience may range from simple relaxation to increased inner awareness, or advance to a sense of pure bliss in the transpersonal dimension. Underlying this practice is the philosophy that the therapist's assistance in the client energy field will help to facilitate and balance energy flow to the area that is most in need of change (Slater, 1995). Thus, the client may obtain relief from physical or emotional pain, release a long-held conflict, think more clearly, or connect with his transpersonal guidance as part of the healing. The facilitator's supportive approach is different from hypnotherapy or self-directed meditation, although outcomes, such as delving into deeper aspects of the subconscious, may be similar.

Another major difference among the three modalities seems to be in purpose and emphasis. Practitioners of hypnotherapy can attest to the effectiveness of their modality in resolving serious emotional distress that is not amenable to cognitive approaches. The focus in hypnotherapy, however, is on pathology and helping the client to work through complex issues while in an altered state. This is distinguished from the spontaneous insights that emerge in an energy-mediated session in which the client seems to bring together his own right and left brain functions for new synthesis. Meditation, similarly, may cause issues to come into one's awareness—awareness is the beginning of all healing—but meditation by itself does not attempt resolution of long-held problems.

The most important difference among these methods is the sense of personal empowerment that clients experience either with meditation or energetic approaches. As clients move toward high-level wellness on their own, they develop self-confidence and personal strength. In hypnotherapy, the control is in the hands of the practitioner who can, if skilled, be an invaluable ally. In the hands of a less skilled or self-seeking operator, the client can become more confused and dependent. For those clients who do not want to take responsibility for all their personal choices, the idea of having someone else direct their lives can be tempting—and full of hazards.

In a nutshell, it is clear that each modality has specific gifts to offer those seeking self-understanding. Meditation connects clients to the inner self most directly; energy-oriented healing gives useful tools for self-empowerment and self-healing; and hypnotherapy connects one to a therapist who hopefully has the knowledge and skill to encourage the use of inner strengths as quickly as possible. It is clear that the holistic framework espouses psychological independence, a willingness to learn from physical and emotional *dis-ease*, and to find the unique path toward resolution. At its finest, the holistic view connects clients to the inner healer and the inherent wisdom within.

The following table further differentiates the three modalities based on the authors' experience. It delineates the major emphasis of each modality, the view of problem resolution, the learning styles involved, the client's sense of control of the experience, the levels of nonordinary consciousness accessed, and the similar outcomes.

Development of a Code of Ethics

From our discussion it is clear that each practitioner needs to evolve a personal code of ethics, while honoring professional guidelines that encompass his or her practice. For energy-oriented healing, special considerations that deal with nonordinary states of consciousness and the concerns we have discussed are included. The challenge of defining the standards of care and code of ethics need to be addressed by the many energy-oriented healers that are currently studying and developing their professional practices of this very young art and science. As a sample, we offer the Code of Ethics for Energy Healers, developed by HAPPEN, in Appendix D.

TABLE 15.1   COMPARISON OF THREE MODALITIES

MODALITY	MEDITATION	HYPNOTHERAPY	ENERGY HEALING
Major Purpose	Seeking personal control of the mind, clarity, concentration	Bring new resolutions to past trauma	Personal development for self-healing, intuitive sensing
View of Problem	Lack of inner knowledge and self-awareness	Psychopathology related to subconscious material	Seeking high level wellness through self-awareness
Problem Solution	Independent seeking, mastery of breath and thought	Therapist devises solution, gives suggestions	Learner finds own solutions, symptoms seen as clues
Learning Style	Meditator works at own pace, daily or sporadically	Client depends on operator/therapist	Connection to one's Higher Self, through relaxation
Control of the Experience	Active, by the meditator	Passive, client allows the therapist to lead	Active, in the client's control with support from therapist
Level of Altered State of Consciousness	Light altered state of consciousness, relaxed	Deep trance, minimal talking	Light to moderate trance, relaxed and alert, active use of imagery
Outcome of Process	Mental clarity, sense of personal truth	Insight, integration of dissociated parts	Connecting to personal truth, self-learning, transpersonal dimension

SUMMARY

In all therapies, the helper's skill involves knowing how to help the client chart a course in the unique territory of the inner psyche without imposing her own limitations or fears. This skill, however, must be further advanced as one prepares for an ethical practice of multidimensional healing. The experience of energy healing is enhanced not so much by what the healer does but by who she is, the very essence of her being that is brought to life through the clarity of her energy field. The field becomes the healer's instrument for facilitating the client's transformation.

REFERENCES

American Association for Marriage and Family Therapy. *Code of Ethics,* August, 1991.

American Psychiatric Association, "APA issues statement on memories of sexual abuse." *Psychiatric Times.* February, 1994, p. 26.

American Psychological Association. *Ethical Principles of Psychologists and Code of Conduct.* 1989.

Brennan, B. *Hands of Light.* New York: Bantam Books.

Ethical agreements for holotropic breathwork practitioners. *The Inner Door.* Santa Cruz, CA: Association for Holotropic Breathwork International, August, 1994.

Ethical *Guidelines for Feminist Therapists.* Boulder, CO: The Feminist Therapy Institute, 1991.

Leadbeater, C. *Thought Forms.* Wheaton, IL: Theosophical Publishing House, 1980.

Manning, R. *Speaking From the Heart: A Feminist Perspective on Ethics.* Lanham, MD: Rowman & Littlefield Publishers, Inc., 1992, p. xiv.

National Association for Music Therapy. *Code of Ethics.* 1992.

Remen, R. N. "On defining spirit." *Noetic Sciences Review.* Autumn, 1988, p. 63.

Ross., C. "Trauma memories and dissociative identity disorder." *Highlights.* 17:1, May, 1995, p. 16–17.

Slater, V. "Toward an understanding of energetic healing, part 2." *Journal of Holistic Nursing,* Vol. 13:3, September, 1995, p. 225–238.

Taylor, K. *The Ethics of Caring.* Santa Cruz, CA: Hanford Mead Publishe ˙ 1995.

Walsh, R. "Phenomenological mapping: A method for describing and comparing states of consciousness." *Journal of Transpersonal Psychology,* Vol. 27:1, 1995, p. 25–56.

Whitfield, C. *Boundaries and Relationships.* Deerfield Beach, FL: Health Communications, Inc., 1993.

Yapko, M. D. *Suggestions of Abuse.* New York: Simon & Schuster, 1994.

16

THE DEEPENING
PRACTICE OF
HEART-CENTERED
CONSCIOUSNESS

Thus far, we have made a beginning exploration of the many intriguing possibilities associated with the use of energy principles for emotional healing. It is an open-ended exploration that will hopefully stimulate discussion, development, research, application, and further refinement in many professional communities. Although many therapists may have already used energy concepts intuitively, in this volume we have attempted to make energy healing explicit within the broader fabric of holistic philosophy.

It remains, then, for us to consider ways of further clarifying and validating this approach to facilitate the use of energetic concepts in counseling and personal growth endeavors. We now explore the need for research, describe our vision of transformational pathways to wholeness, and conclude by affirming the expanded view of healing set forth in the first chapter.

THE NEED FOR RESEARCH

It goes without saying that dissemination of this information and its application in the diverse practices of humanistic therapies requires research to support and validate the results shown in the individual case examples we have cited. Because multidimensional healing is a complex event, traditional research methods requiring exact replication and double blind studies may be too limiting to be appropriate. The variables leading to psychospiritual integration are immense when we consider the thousands of influences that affect the energy field of the client, let alone those impacting the field of the healer. We might concur, after viewing the case presentations in this book, that each healing example represents a unique and unrepeatable event. The exact circumstances that made new insights possible were truly multidimensional in nature.

Currently, popular research traditions in the social sciences limit research design to a very small number of variables. This requires that more subjective factors, such as perceived emotional support and remembered past history, are selectively ignored. It is a seeming paradox that many clients are seeking alternative healing modalities and sensing their own energy fields at a time when scientific explorations have become more narrow and reductionist in focus. This phenomenon suggests not that we ignore the experiences of such clients but rather that we find new ways of conceptualizing and broadening research design.

Waiting until total, indisputable evidence supports common sense about what is harmful or helpful can create an enormous time gap. This lag in time leaves us open to unnecessary loss and suffering. Consider, for example, the more than twenty years that were needed to convincingly document the effects of smoking and second-hand smoke on the body. Long before the evidence was conclusive, common sense and medical information let us know that cigarette smoking was a serious health hazard. Today's sophisticated, empowered health care consumers are interested in complementary approaches and self-care, even when difficult to measure objectively. The intelligent consumer desires the best care that is available, including the unconventional. Therefore, our concepts of research design must expand to assess multidimensional changes and meet the demands of the changing face of health care.

How, indeed, could we objectively measure an individual's internal experience of being assisted through energy field balancing? Should we simply ignore these valuable inner experiences that lead to new perceptions and insights? Abraham Maslow, recognized co-founder of humanistic and transpersonal psychology movements exhorts us: "If there is any primary rule of science, it is . . . acceptance of the obligation to acknowledge and describe all of reality . . . even that which it cannot understand or explain, and that for which no theory exists, that which cannot be measured, predicted, controlled, or ordered. . . ." (Maslow, 1966).

Larry Dossey, leading medical philosopher of the holistic paradigm and editor of the highly acclaimed new journal *Alternative Therapies*, suggests a path out of this conundrum. "Should healers be expected to heal on each and every attempt, as skeptics demand?" he asks (1995, p. 79). "We do not make this demand of other human abilities. If an athlete runs a 4-minute mile on one occasion, we do not require that he repeat the achievement on every successive attempt in order to prove that the initial accomplishment was valid." Running a 4-minute mile is a unique human achievement that is publicly acknowledged without ever requiring a repeated demonstration by the same runner. Consciousness-based therapies, such as the energy healing work we have described, could be viewed in the same manner. Each healing event is unique and essentially unrepeatable. However, we can study the phenomena observed and draw conclusions about specific interventions and intents on the part of the helper that facilitate the probability of change.

Multidimensional healing may best be examined by phenomenological research methods (Giorgi, 1985). Within this method, each person's experience is explored in detail, providing in-depth data that can be compared with new and developing insights. Phenomenological research has been used successfully in many dissertations within the holistic science of nursing, allowing the addition of personal reflection to other measurable data. For example, Mabbett described caregivers who maintained high levels of vitality and she was able to deduce the six major components of vitality in the workplace from a relatively small sample of health care professionals (Mabbett, 1989). This research allowed her to generate a model for maintaining caregiver vitality in a variety of settings (Hover-Kramer, Mabbett, and Shames, 1996).

Since energy-related interventions have so many variables and a wide range of effects, phenomenological research may be the best avenue for expanding our data base. The kinds of human emotional needs we have considered in this book deserve our full exploration and scientific acumen. Healthy skepticism, a quality both authors endorse and encourage in others, requires a willingness to stay open-minded to the phenomena that clients report.

TRANSFORMATIONAL PATHWAYS TO WHOLENESS

Energy healing is one of the many pathways that lead to personal transformation—change that is pervasive and lasting which resonates within the farther reaches of human consciousness. Inherent in the energy healing process are elements not usually addressed in therapy: sensing the vital life force through the human energy field; exploring identity beyond the personal ego; connecting with boundless consciousness; and working with the focused intentionality of the healer. As the client seeks understanding of his traumatic past or current conflicts, the energy therapist can help to pinpoint the exact area in the energy field associated with the embedded, difficult material. This, then, allows the client to identify issues related to the affected energy centers and the layers of the field. Working at his own pace, the client can address the energetic constriction, transform the turbulence, and fill in the gaps of missing knowledge or emotional support.

Throughout the process, the therapist works within the client's frame of reference while simultaneously respecting his internal states. The metaphors of excision, or exorcism, might fit the actual discharge of the conflicted, disturbed material, but would be used only if they had meaning for the client. The responsibility for growth and the pace of learning rests entirely with the client and his sense of safety and readiness. As we have illustrated, the insights that grow out of illusion-shattering experiences can lead to direct knowing (called *gnosis* by the Greeks). Gnosis brings a sense of inner truth that resonates throughout the various dimensions of the client's being to bring about new integration and wholeness. For example, the client no longer thinks or believes that he is connected to the Infinite. He *knows* it.

The metaphor of an overloaded computer disk comes to mind in describing the internal state of many clients entering psychotherapy. As old, overloading patterns are released, similar to the dumping of excessive material from the disk, there is room for a tremendous influx of new energy, new thought, and new interconnections within the psyche.

Transformation, then, becomes visible in one's entire approach to life: the distracted, overloaded mind becomes focused; old rules become part of new choices; limited thinking reaches to unlimited opportunities; worry about the past or future translates into being fully in the present; external locus of control moves to an internal sense of power; and the ultimate fear of death transmutes into curiosity about the immortal nature of the soul.

LIVING WITH THE EXPANDED VIEW OF HEALING

We have come full circle in describing our expanded view of healing by way of directed human consciousness, for psychotherapy, and self-care. The holistic paradigm gives us a springboard for exploring all the dimensions of human experience, physical functioning, emotional sensing, mental patterning, and spiritual connecting. As we conceptualize the human energy field, we have a specific framework for facilitating the client's process.

Throughout energy work, we remember healing is the gift of grace: not by our own power, but by alignment with the Universal Energies. The client's higher resources allows healing to becomes possible. The work of the healer, teacher, or facilitator is simply to create the circumstances for the divine nature of the individual to flow to its higher vibrational pattern, and for the elevated forces within to come to the forefront.

We have suggested that the metaphor of centering with the open heart is a tool that is available to all of us, whether client or healer. Turning the light of this caring towards others, we can become agents for their change and transformation. Turning the light of this caring within ourselves, we access our own inner healer.

Our human energy field and its expanding consciousness persists and continues to develop beyond the present physical lifetime in the same way that the mind awakens in the morning after a dream.

IN CONCLUSION . . .

What the mind can only guess,
Or grasp in piecemeal fashion,

The intuitive knows
Without question.
It soars like an eagle
Above the fragmented self
And lifts to the mystery,
The unknown, the unnamable,
Beyond limits of time and space
To connect with the timeless,
Eternal
And whole.

—DHK

REFERENCES

Dossey, L. "How should alternative therapies be evaluated?" *Alternative Therapies in Health and Medicine.* May, 1995, I:2, p. 6–10, 79–85.

Giorgi, A. *Psychology as a Human Science: A Phomenologically Based Approach.* New York: Harper & Row, 1985.

Hover-Kramer, D., Mabbett, P., and Shames, K. H. "Vitality for caregivers." *Holistic Nursing Practice.* January, 1996, Vol. 10:2, p. 38–48.

Mabbett. P. *Depletion vs. Regenerative Responses Among Institutional Caregivers: A Phenomenological Investigation.* Del Mar, CA: University for Humanistic Studies, 1989, Unpublished Dissertation.

Maslow, A. *The Psychology of Science.* New York: Harper & Row, 1966.

LIST OF EXERCISES GIVEN IN THIS BOOK

SELECTED PROGRAMS IN ENERGY HEALING

Appendix

A

Barbara Brennan School of Healing
P.O. Box 2005
East Hampton, NY 11937
(516) 329-0951

Core Energetics
Institute of Core Energetics
115 E. 23rd Street
New York, NY 10010
(212) 982-9637

Healing Light Center Church
Rev. Rosalyn L. Bruyere
261 East Alegria #12
Sierra Madre, CA 91024
(818) 306-2170

Healing Touch
Colorado Center for Healing Touch
198 Union Boulevard, Suite 210
Lakewood, CO 80228
(303) 989-0581

Leonard Laskow's Healing with Love Foundation
Leonard Laskow, M.D.
20 Sunnyside Avenue, #334
Mill Valley, CA 94941
(800) 381-0747

Nirvana School of Enlightenment™
Mary Bell, RNC
7127 E. Becker Lane, Suite 157
Scottsdale, AZ 85254
(602) 230-5249

Nurse Healers–Professional Associates, Inc.
Janet Ziegler, R.N., M.N.
c/o NH-PA, Inc.
P.O. Box 444
Allison Park, PA 15101-0444
(412) 355-8476

School of Enlightenment and Healing
Dr. Michael Mamas
P.O. Box 9087
San Diego, CA 92169
(619) 272-4147

Shen Therapy
International Shen Therapy Association
P.O. Box 801
Edmonds, WA 98020
(206) 298-9468

Transformational Pathways
HAPPEN (Holistic Alliance of Professional Practitioners,
 Entrepreneurs, and Networkers, Inc.)
1031 NW 6 Street, Suite F-1
Gainesville, FL 32601
(352) 337-1185

___

ENERGY- RELATED PROGRAMS, THERAPIES, AND ORGANIZATIONS

We have included a partial listing of energy-related therapies and organizations. Many others can be located in individual communities.

Guided Imagery

Academy for Guided Imagery (AGI)
P.O. Box 2070
Mill Valley, CA. 94941
(800) 726-2070

Nurses' Certificate Program in Interactive Imagery
Beyond Ordinary Nursing
P.O. Box 8177
Foster City, CA 94404-3004
(415) 570-6157

Holistic Nursing

American Holistic Nurses Association
4101 Lake Boone Trail, Suite 201
Raleigh, NC 27607
(919) 787-5181

Humanistic Psychology

Association for Humanistic Psychology
45 Franklin Street, Suite 315
San Francisco, CA 94502
(415) 864-8850

Massage Therapy

American Massage Therapy Association
820 Davis Street, Suite 100
Evanston, IL 60201-4444
(708) 864-0123

National Association of Nurse Massage Therapists
Randy Bryson, R.N.
1720 Willow Creek Circle
Eugene OR 97402
(541) 485-7372

Associated Bodyworkers and Massage Professionals
28677 Buffalo Park
Evergreen, CO 80439-7347
(303) 674-8478

Oriental Bodywork

American Oriental Bodywork Therapy Association
6801 Jericho Turnpike
Syosset, NY 11791
(516) 365-0808

Jin Shin Jyutsu
8719 E. San Alberto
Scottsdale, AZ 85258
(602) 998-9331

Polarity Therapy

American Polarity Therapy Association
2888 Bluff Street, Suite 149
Boulder, CO. 80301
(303) 545-2080

Reflexology

American Reflexology Certification Board
P.O. Box 620607
Littleton, CO 80162
(303) 933-6921

Reiki

American International Reiki Association
2210 Wilshire Boulevard, #831
Santa Monica, CA 90403
(310) 788-1821

American Reiki Master Association
Box 130
Lake City, FL 32056
(904) 755-9638

Reiki Alliance
P.O. Box 41
Cataldo, ID 83810
(208) 682-3535

Somatic Therapies

DC Guild of Body-Psychotherapists
1111 Bonifant Street, Suite 201
Silver Springs, MD 20910
(301) 589-0390

Federation of Therapeutic Massage, Bodywork, & Somatic
 Practices Organizations
820 Davis Street, #100
Evanston, IL. 60201-4444
(708) 864-0123

International Center for Release and Integration
450 Hillside Avenue
Mill Valley, CA 94941
(415) 383-4017

Rosen Method Bodywork
The Berkeley Center
825 Bancroft Way
Berkeley, CA 94710
(510) 845-6606

Trager Institute
21 Locust Avenue
Mill Valley, CA 94941-2806
(415) 388-2688

Touch for Health® Association
3223 Washington Blvd., Suite 201
Marina del Rey, CA 90292
(800) 466-8342

Subtle Energy Medicine

International Society for the Study of Subtle Energies/Energy
 Medicine
356 Golden Circle
Golden, CO 80403
(303) 278-2228

Transpersonal Psychology

Association for Transpersonal Psychology
P.O. Box 3049
Stanford, CA 94309
(415) 327-2066

SAMPLE PSYCHOENERGETIC INTAKE SHEET

Date_____

Identifying Data

Name _____Telephone #_____

Address _____Zip _____

Profession _____

Physical Status

Presenting Symptoms _____

Current Medications _____

Pertinent History_____

Emotional Status

Current Stress in Personal and Professional Life_____

Predominant Emotion_____

How Would Client Rate Emotional Health?_____

Current Sources of Pleasure _____

Mental Status

Predominant Thought Patterns _____

How Would Client Rate Mental Health?_____

Meditation Practice _____

Frequency/Effectiveness _____

Spiritual Awareness

Does Client Feel Connected to a Higher Power? _____

How Does this Assist? _____

Energetic Assessment

Areas of Energy Field Disturbance/Imbalance _____

Condition of the Major Energy Centers _____

Intuitive Perceptions_____

Appendix

C | SAMPLE INFORMED CONSENT FORM

I understand that Energy Healing is a complementary modality that in no way substitutes for appropriate medical intervention, body therapy, or other forms of psychotherapy. I also understand that my practitioner will make suggestions for my self-care and referrals based on wide experience.

I recognize that there is a close working partnership between me and my therapist that requires me to share my ideas, perceptions, and opinions readily. In this manner any misunderstandings can be cleared up immediately.

I hold my therapist harmless from any liability for my physical condition and state of mind. Although no harmful effects have been noted in any of the research literature, I understand that my energy field is unique and may respond in unique ways to energetic interventions. Internal changes in self-esteem and thinking patterns have been noted with energy healing and may constitute a risk or benefit, depending on my perception.

I further understand that there are numerous benefits possible in this type of healing work, such as diminished pain sensation, increased relaxation, relief from anxiety, and enhanced sense of well-being. I agree to take full responsibility for my self care in the physical, emotional, and mental dimensions of my life as much as possible.

Signed _____

Printed Name _____

Date _____

Appendix

D CODE OF ETHICS FOR TRANSFORMATIONAL HEALERS

(as developed by Holistic Alliance of Professional Practitioners, Entrepreneurs, and Networkers, Inc. [HAPPEN] 1996.)

Standard of Ethical Consideration #1 (in Relation to Self):

Transformational Healers shall maintain integrity of their personal transformational field.

Standards of Practice

A. Transformational Healers have growing and sensitive awareness of their personal issues in physical/emotional/ mental/spiritual dimensions of their transformational field.

B. Transformational Healers seek appropriate help for physical/emotional/mental/spiritual issues as soon as they become aware of their personal need.

C. Transformational Healers ultimately trust their own inner wisdom, based on information and feedback from the client's field.

D. Transformational Healers commit to independent thinking, thus avoiding overinvolvement/overattachment with anyone else's point of view.

Standard of Ethical Consideration #2:
(in Relation to Clients)

Transformational Healers consider the client's needs in the physical/ emotional/mental/spiritual realms as the priority when providing care.

Standards of Practice

   A. Transformational Healers set their intent for the highest good of the client, relinquishing any attachments, personal agendas, or need for specific outcomes.

   B. Transformational Healers ensure that their own sense of personal gratification is derived from sources other than the client.

   C. Transformational Healers shall provide highest quality of care possible based on their theory and knowledge base.

   D. Transformational Healers continually evaluate client outcomes and revise plan of care accordingly.

Standard of Ethical Consideration #3
(in Relation to Colleagues)

Transformational Healers treat their colleagues with respect and honor.

Standards of Practice

   A. Transformational Healers avoid public discussion of differences of opinion.

   B. Transformational Healers discuss differences of opinion directly with the person involved; no third party conversations.

   C. If direct discussion does not bring resolution, Transformational Healers seek arbitration/mediation, beginning with local resources then state, regional, or national as deemed necessary for resolution.

Standard of Ethical Consideration #4:
(concerning Referrals and Consultants)

Transformational Healers readily utilize referral and consultant resources to maximize client's well-being.

Standards of Practice

   A. Transformational Healers take responsibility for defining and clarifying their practice to their local professional community.

   B. Transformational Healers collaborate with professionals who refer clients for transformational healing, communicating frequently and returning client to primary caregiver as soon as possible.

C. Transformational Healers identify client needs beyond their scope of practice, referring to appropriate resources as quickly as possible.

D. Transformational Healers establish the concepts of transformational healing within appropriate professional organizations in their local community.

E. Transformational Healers donate a portion of their time for making public contributions to a general awareness of transformational healing practices.

GLOSSARY OF
ENERGY-RELATED TERMS

Acupuncture: The art and science from the ancient Chinese tradition of working with subtle energy flows in the body known as meridians, via specific access centers known as acupuncture points, to restore balance to the human energy system.

Aura: The Human Energy Field (HEF) that surrounds and blends with the physical body which is its densest form. It consists of distinctive layers corresponding to physical, emotional, mental, spiritual and subtle aspects of the multidimensional human being. Also called the *human biofield*.

Balancing: Term referring to the realignment of the HEF to its natural highest function and organization.

Centering: The process of focusing one's intention to be fully present and responsive to one's client by setting aside personal mental, emotional, or physical issues for the moment.

Chakra: Sanskrit word meaning wheel; used to describe the human energy centers.

Ch'i: Chinese term for energy or vital life force that acts as nourishing subtle energy circulating through the acupuncture meridians and human energy system. Also called *prana, qi,* or *ki*.

Clairaudience: The ability to hear words, sounds, or rhythms with intuitive higher sense perception.

Clairsentience: The ability to use the intuitive aspect of touch to detect subtle temperature changes, textures, vibrations, or other kinesthetic phenomena.

Clairvoyance: The ability to see colors, shapes, or images with intuitive higher sense perception. In the French language, it literally means "clear seeing."

Clearing: The therapist's small or large hand movements in the HEF that facilitate release of energy blockage. Synonymous with discharging, releasing, unforming, letting go, smoothing, and unruffling.

Consciousness: The primary human essence, the continuing sense of self or "I," that is evident in waking awareness as well as in altered states, such as centering, meditation, dreams, trance, or near-death experiences.

Energy Blockage: A general term referring to the interruption or constriction of the natural flow patterns in the human energy system. May refer to a closed or diminished energy center or asymmetry in the energy field.

Energy Center: A specific center of consciousness in the human energy system that allows for the inflow of energy from the Universal Energy Field as well as for outflow from the individual's energy field. In relation to the physical body, the energy centers convert subtle energy into chemical, hormonal, and cellular changes. There are 7 major energy centers in relation to the spine and many minor centers at bone articulations in the palms of the hands and at the soles of the feet. Also called *Chakra.*

Energy Healing: Healing interventions that address releasing of energetic blockage or imbalance followed by repatterning, balancing, and aligning of the Human Energy Field to higher levels of functioning.

Healing: The ongoing evolution toward higher levels of functioning in the multidimensional human being.

Holistic Health: An integrated approach to human well-being that combines attention to the physical, emotional, mental, and spiritual aspects of the individual in the context of his environment.

Hologram: The three-dimensional image created by the interference pattern of two interacting laser beams. Any part of the hologram contains the information of the whole. The human mind appears to function as a hologram, allowing a single word or image to generate a whole complex of inner experiences.

Human Energy System: The entire interactive dynamic of human subtle energies, consisting of the energy centers, the multidimensional field, the meridians, and the acupuncture points.

Grounding: Connecting to the earth and earth's energy field to calm the mind and focus one's inner flow of energy,

Imagery: Broad concept that involves thoughts, feelings, and sensations associated with a symbolic representation. The symbols may be generated from all of the senses: visual, auditory, kinesthetic, taste, or smell.

Intention: Holding one's inner awareness and focus for accomplishing a specific action; being fully present in the moment.

Kundalini: In Yogic philosophy, the creative energy of spiritual illumination that is stored at the base of the spine. As the individual progresses in his path of awareness, the kundalini begins to flow upward and gently activate the higher centers of consciousness. Forcing the process too quickly may cause uncomfortable vibrations or spasms known as *kryas.*

Meridians: The subtle energy flow lines that course through the human body. According to Oriental philosophies, these flows correspond to specific organs and systems.

Modulation of Energy: The therapist's gentle holding movements that facilitate energetic balancing or filling in depleted parts of the HEF. Synonymous with transferring energy from the universal field, transforming, and repatterning.

Prana: East Indian word for vital life force, or *ch'i. Pranayama* is the ongoing study and meditation to activate prana.

Psychoenergetic Healing: A specific form of healing practice that interrelates psychological insights with energetic principles.

Psychoneuroimmunology (PNI):   Medical term for the evolving discipline that studies the interaction between body and mind, the emotions, neurotransmitters, and the immune system to understand illness and facilitate well-being.

Relaxation Response: Term coined by Dr. H. Benson to refer to the systemic responses and restorative results of activating the parasympathetic nervous system through meditative or centering practices.

Transpersonal: Term coined by Drs. Maslow, Sutich, and Grof to describe the psychological realm beyond the personal, and reaching to the wider, spiritual dimension of human experience.

Universal Energy Field (UEF):   The infinite resource of energy that surrounds and penetrates all aspects of the universe. Other terms include Source, All that Is, The Absolute, The Ground of Being, Creative Spirit, Nonlocal Mind, and Good Orderly Direction.

Unruffling: Term coined by Dr. D. Krieger to suggest the clearing of a ruffled or turbulent area in the HEF.

Sensitive: A person who is able to use intuitive higher sense perception to assess the human energy system and other subtle energies.

INDEX